Restructuring Chronic Illness Management

Jon B. Christianson
Ruth A. Taylor
David J. Knutson

Restructuring Chronic Illness Management

Best Practices and Innovations in Team-Based Treatment

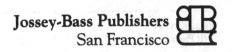

Jossey-Bass Publishers
San Francisco

Substantial discounts on bulk quantities of Jossey-Bass books are available to corporations, professional associations, and other organizations. For details and discount information, contact the special sales department at Jossey-Bass Inc., Publishers (415) 433–1740; Fax (800) 605–2665.

For sales outside the United States, please contact your local Simon & Schuster International Office.

Jossey-Bass Web address: http://www.josseybass.com

Library of Congress Cataloging-in-Publication Data
Christianson, Jon B.
    Restructuring chronic illness management : best practices and innovations in team-based treatment / Jon B. Christianson, Ruth A. Taylor, David J. Knutson. — 1st ed.
        p.   cm.
    Includes bibliographical references and index.
    ISBN 978-0-470-63102-7
    1. Chronic diseases—Treatment.   2. Chronic diseases—Treatment—Economic aspects.   3. Health planning.   4. Health care teams.
5. Medical protocols.   I. Taylor, Ruth A.   II. Knutson, David J.
    [DNLM: 1. Chronic Disease—therapy.   2. Patient Care Planning—organization & administration.   3. Patient Care Team.   4. Models, Organizational.   WT 500 C555r 1998]
RA644.5.C466   1998
616'.044—dc21
DNLM/DLC
for Library of Congress   97-46162
                                                                                        CIP

FIRST EDITION
HB *Printing*   10 9 8 7 6 5 4 3 2 1

Contents

List of Tables and Figures

Tables

Figures

Preface

Almost half of America's noninstitutionalized population now suffers from some form of chronic illness, and this proportion is likely to increase as the population ages. The average cost of treating individuals with chronic illnesses is three times the cost of care for others and is growing rapidly. These facts underscore the pressures on health care delivery systems to develop and implement new approaches for treating chronic illnesses. These innovative approaches must improve patient outcomes while conserving increasingly scarce treatment resources.

The existing literature contains descriptions and evaluations of various innovative approaches to chronic illness management, but it is relatively silent on the organizational and financial issues that can arise when these models are implemented in real-world settings. Yet these issues are likely to be substantial, because virtually any restructuring in the treatment of chronic illnesses is likely to challenge cultural norms and generate significant stakeholder resistance within health care organizations.

This book is based on the premise that health care organizations must pay attention to organizational and financial issues, as well as clinical ones, when implementing new approaches to the treatment of chronic illnesses. The book's purpose is to assist decision makers in health care organizations as they attempt to transform promising ideas for chronic illness treatment into operational programs.

The book's structure reflects this purpose. It begins with a discussion of the published literature, augments this with the experiences of operational programs, proposes a specific model that synthesizes these findings, and provides a tool that organizations can use when planning and implementing this or similar models.

The first two chapters discuss the nature of chronic illness, along with the challenges that its treatment poses for the health care system. The potential for a team approach to the treatment of chronic illness is also discussed.

Chapter Three reviews the published literature about the characteristics and effectiveness of new treatment approaches for specific chronic illnesses. The models described in these research studies have several common features that can form the basis for restructuring chronic illness treatment within health care organizations. Issues of organization and implementation are seldom addressed in the studies, however, except as post hoc explanations of why particular treatment approaches were not as effective as anticipated. Chapters Four and Five address these issues, drawing primarily on literature about the design and functioning of work groups.

Although the published literature on both clinical and organizational issues provides important and useful guidance on the reorganization of chronic illness treatment, examining the experience of ongoing programs can yield additional insights. Chapter Six describes eight different chronic illness management efforts. These include relatively small-scale initiatives aimed at delivering care more effectively to targeted groups of patients, as well as major attempts to revamp care processes in large managed care organizations. Together, these program descriptions illustrate how chronic illness management initiatives are being implemented.

To explore operational issues relating to these programs even further, we convened a panel of program representatives. Chapter Seven presents the set of principles that the panel developed for chronic illness management, along with panel members' edited comments.

Chapter Eight describes a prototypical chronic illness management model. This model reflects the lessons drawn from the published literature (Chapters Two through Five), the experience of ongoing programs (Chapter Six), and the principles outlined in Chapter Seven. Critical issues relating to model design and implementation in actual organizational settings also are discussed in this chapter.

The final chapter gives health care organizations a framework for assessing their own readiness to change. This framework should help them think systematically about implementation and operational issues as they plan to restructure chronic illness treatment. This framework is further developed in the form of an assessment tool, which appears in the Appendix.

Institute for Research and Education   Jon B. Christianson
Minneapolis   Ruth A. Taylor
February 1998   David J. Knutson

Acknowledgments

We are deeply grateful to all of our colleagues whose contributions, advice, experience, and encouragement provided us with a solid foundation for this book. In particular, we thank the following groups.

The National Consensus Panel members, for their expertise and insights into the successes and challenges of developing and implementing new models of care in clinical settings: Donnell Etzwiler, Halsted Holman, Kathleen Loane, Karen Meyer, Mary Pat Paquette, Janice Smith Pigg, Joe Selby, Victor Villagra, and Michael Von Korff.

The Project Advisory Committee members from HealthSystem Minnesota, who provided thoughtful and practical views from both the primary care and specialty perspectives that helped us focus our work: David Abelson, Renner Anderson, Richard Bergenstal, Michael Dukinfield, Eric Schned, William Schoenwetter, and Anthony Woolley.

The Institute for Research and Education and especially James V. Toscano, executive vice president, for his continued encouragement and support of this work.

Elizabeth Fowler and Marjorie Ireland, for their critical review of the literature and concise summaries, which formed the basis of Chapter Three.

Jonathan Weiner and Jinnet Fowles, who read and critiqued the manuscript in its early stage.

Aleta Millette and the administrative support staff in the Health Research Center, for their patience and skill in making numerous revisions to the manuscript.

Finally, we wish to thank Hoechst Marion Roussel, Inc., Merck & Co., Inc., and Rhône-Poulenc Rorer Pharmaceuticals, Inc. Their financial support allowed us to undertake the work that generated this book.

The Authors

Jon B. Christianson received a bachelor's degree in mathematics and economics from St. Olaf College (1968) and a doctorate in economics from the University of Wisconsin-Madison (1974). He teaches courses in managed care and in cost-effectiveness analysis in health care to graduate students at the University of Minnesota, where he is a professor in the Division of Health Services Research and Policy, School of Public Health. Previously, he served on the faculties of the University of Arizona and Montana State University. He has extensive research experience related to the financing and evaluating of medical care. He has authored or coauthored six books and more than one hundred articles in the areas of managed care, long-term care, rural health care, and mental health care, and he has collaborated with health care providers in a variety of practice settings to evaluate new treatment approaches. Currently, he is a member of the editorial boards of *Health Affairs* and *Medical Care Research and Review*. In 1995, he coauthored a paper that won the annual Health Care Research Award of the National Institute for Health Care Management.

Ruth A. Taylor is a project coordinator in the Health Research Center of the Institute for Research and Education in Minneapolis. She earned a bachelor's degree from Valparaiso University (1969). Taylor has extensive experience in program implementation, survey

development, patient advocacy, management of national and local
outcomes studies, and coordination of clinical trials. She is a member of the Institutional Review Board (IRB) for the protection of
human subjects and sits on the Advisory Committee for Health-
System Minnesota's three IRBs. Taylor has been the project manager for the first and second phases of A Collaborative Model of
Chronic Illness Management; that project serves as the basis for
this book.

David J. Knutson is director of the Health Systems Studies Division
at the Institute for Research and Education of HealthSystem
Minnesota. There, in Minneapolis, he conducts research on health
care organization, finance, and policy. He has extensive experience
in health care administration in both the private and public sectors;
he has directed a residential mental health facility, a regional emergency medical services program, and a provider network management for a large HMO. Mr. Knutson has published a number of
articles related to risk-based payment methods, health care con-
sumerism, and clinical outcomes assessment. He has a B.A. in biol-
ogy from Augsburg College in Minneapolis (1969) and is currently
a graduate student at the University of Minnesota.

Restructuring Chronic Illness Management

1

The Challenge of
Managing Chronic Illness
Pressures and Options

A recent issue of the *Journal of the American Medical Association* (Hoffman, Rice, and Sung, 1996) underscored in stark terms the challenge of managing chronic illness. There are now approximately one hundred million people (45 percent of the noninstitutionalized population) in the United States with one or more chronic illnesses. More than $600 billion (in 1990 dollars) is spent annually on their care, including $425 billion in direct medical care expenses. On average, health care costs for individuals with chronic illnesses are three times the costs of the care delivered to others. As the United States's population ages over the next few decades, expenditures for chronic illness care are expected to increase dramatically from this already high level.

One of the most significant challenges now facing the United States health care system is to develop new approaches for managing chronic illness care. These approaches must be clinically appropriate, cost effective, and capable of being implemented in real-world settings. Given the decentralized, private sector orientation of health care delivery in the United States, the pressure to meet this challenge will fall primarily on organized health care systems (Fishman, Von Korff, Lozano, and Itecht, 1997). How should they respond?

Some published studies address the clinical effectiveness of specific chronic illness management models compared with usual

1

practice, but the literature is relatively silent on the organizational and financial issues that can arise in designing and implementing these models. Many models require restructuring care processes in ways that could challenge deeply held beliefs and long-standing cultural norms within health care organizations. These changes can also be financially challenging for organizations, because they often include activities that payers do not typically reimburse (Peterson, 1995). For these reasons, there is likely to be substantial stakeholder resistance within organizations. To surmount this resistance, managerial attention and a commitment of resources will be required (Lumsdon, 1995).

This book is based on the ongoing experience of a health care delivery system—HealthSystem Minnesota—in its attempts to plan for and address these issues. HealthSystem Minnesota consists of a 350-physician multispecialty group practice, a primary care physician network, a 467-bed hospital, a research foundation (the Institute for Research and Education, or IRE), and numerous other programs and specialized treatment centers. It draws most of its patients from managed care organizations, self-insured employers, and Medicare. Its multispecialty group practice attracts large numbers of chronically ill patients who require intensive, ongoing attention. Like other health care organizations across the United States, HealthSystem Minnesota functions in a world of financial limitations, organizational constraints, media pressures, purchaser exhortations to "do more with less," and consumer perceptions that, increasingly, medical care is more about "curing" than "caring."

In 1994, the IRE at HealthSystem Minnesota began to explore alternative models for treating chronic illnesses. Its goal was to identify or develop a model, or models, that could improve quality of care and patient satisfaction. It also was important that the model, or models, could be implemented in real-world settings and could control costs, a major concern of purchasers.

Staff at the IRE began by reviewing the clinical and management literature. In addition, they canvassed colleagues and notable experts in the area of chronic illness to identify innovative models that care systems were currently implementing. They then assembled a panel of experts and asked them to discuss their experiences with chronic illness management and to distill a set of principles for model development. This book reports the results of this process. Because it reflects the experience of a community-based health care delivery system in rethinking chronic illness management, it addresses not only conceptual issues but also operational concerns.

Definitions of Chronic Illness

Historically, it has been common to define *chronic illness* as any condition that is not acute. With acute illnesses, the patient has been considered cured with the removal of an agent or disease and with the patient's return to normal functioning (Pawlson, 1994). Medical intervention has been seen as appropriate if it produces this type of cure. Any situation that does not fit this paradigm has been called *nonacute*, or *chronic*.

More recently, attempts have been made to develop more precise definitions of *chronic illness*. For example, Jennings, Callahan, and Caplan (1988, p. 4) suggest that "chronic illness may be defined as a condition that lasts for a substantial period of time or has sequelae that are debilitating for a long period of time. It is also commonly defined as a condition that interferes with daily functioning for more than three months in a year, causes hospitalization for thirty days or more per year, or (at the time of diagnosis) is likely to do either of these." In this statement, the attempt to combine a very general concept with specific indicators suggests that chronic illness may be more easily defined by example than in the abstract. In fact, these authors observe that "chronic illness includes a very broad spectrum of diseases that differ significantly from one another in their underlying causes, modes of treatment, symptoms, and effects on a person's life and activity" (p. 4).

There have been several attempts in the literature to divide this "broad spectrum of diseases" into subcategories that make conceptually or clinically useful distinctions among conditions. One such categorization scheme, as proposed by Conrad (1987), separates chronic illnesses into three groups: "lived-with illnesses," "mortal illnesses," and "at-risk illnesses." Individuals must "adapt to and learn to live with" the first type—the lived-with illnesses—but they are not usually life-threatening (p. 24). They include diseases such as diabetes, asthma, arthritis, and epilepsy. Conrad groups them together because, "while these illnesses have different symptoms and manifestations, the problems that people must deal with and the strategies they develop may be quite similar" (p. 24).

Unlike lived-with conditions, mortal illnesses (such as cancer and cardiovascular diseases) are clearly life-threatening. In describing conditions in this category, Conrad notes that "these illnesses take people out of their everyday life (roles) and present them with both symptoms and a threat of death. While there is no 'cure' for most lived-with illness, some forms of mortal illness can be cured or at least remitted in some people" (p. 25).

In contrast to both of these types of chronic illness, the important feature of at-risk illness "is not the illness per se but the risk of illness" (p. 25). The most important example in this category is probably hypertension, but an expanded conceptualization would include environmental contaminants and diseases linked to heredity.

Clearly, these categories are not mutually exclusive, as Conrad acknowledges: "Many illnesses have severe and mild forms and different stages or exacerbations which would place them in different categories. For example, heart disease may be a 'mortal' illness at one point and an 'at-risk' or 'lived-with' illness at another. While most forms of diabetes could be depicted as a 'lived-with' illness, many people with diabetes are also 'at-risk' for ESRD, blindness, or limb disorders and amputations" (p. 26). In this book, the term *chronic illness* will refer to lived-with chronic illnesses, in Conrad's terminology, and to at-risk illnesses to a lesser extent. In discussing the clinical literature, the book will focus more narrowly on five chronic illnesses: arthritis, asthma, diabetes, hypertension, and stable coronary artery disease.

Pressures for Change

It is important for clinicians, researchers, policymakers, pharmaceutical companies, and payers to rethink the delivery and reimbursement of care for individuals with chronic illness. From a clinical point of view, it is increasingly recognized that "intensive, high technology treatment oriented toward cure and full restoration of function, which has provided the dominant orientation for much of medicine in recent years, is usually inappropriate to the needs and problems of the chronically ill" (Jennings, Callahan, and Caplan, 1988, p. 2). Hoffman and Rice (1996) agree with this assessment. They believe that "from the chronic care perspective, key elements of our current 'system' of care—its priorities, allocation of resources, training of professionals, and the incentives inherent in its financing—appear out of kilter and sometimes simply dysfunctional" (p. 11).

This recognition is reflected in the clinical literature by a number of articles describing trial programs, or components of programs, for the management of specific chronic conditions. (We describe some of these programs in Chapter Three.) This literature typically emphasizes the need to involve nonphysician health care workers, the patient, and the patient's family in the ongoing treatment of a chronic illness (Wagner, Austin, and Von Korff, 1996). These topics receive relatively less attention in the treatment of acute illness. This new perspective is reflected in the general policy discussion about the roles of primary care and specialist physicians, as well as in the widespread perception that there are too many specialists

(Cunningham, 1995; Christakis, Jacobs, and Messikomer, 1994; Greenwald and others, 1984).

Public and private sector payers have focused on the need to create financial incentives (by restructuring payments to providers) that encourage cost-effective approaches to the treatment of chronic conditions. In this vein, there is a burgeoning literature on the "risk-adjustment" of capitated payments to managed care organizations (for example, Newhouse, 1994). The premise of this literature is that purchasers need to develop reimbursement mechanisms that do not penalize health care organizations financially for enrolling a disproportionate number of chronically ill individuals. Instead, these reimbursement systems would give health care organizations incentives to deliver care efficiently to those with chronic illnesses.

In addition to their concern about payment issues, purchasers in some communities are collaborating with providers in implementing treatment guidelines for chronic illnesses (Defino, 1995). Although these guidelines describe what *ought* to be done in treating specific patients with chronic illnesses, they typically say little about *how* to do it (Schellevis and others, 1994). This places the burden on health care organizations to develop treatment models that are both cost effective and consistent with such guidelines for chronic illness treatment.

The search for cost-effective approaches to the management of chronic illness has underscored the health educator's potential importance in the treatment process. Educating the patient is seen as cost effective because "free" patient time can be substituted for clinician time. This requires teaching the patient about the disease, though, and possibly training the patient to perform specific functions (Speedling and Rose, 1985; Brody, 1980; McCann and Blossom, 1990; Russell and Roter, 1993). The literature on patient education and training programs has expanded in response to these demands (for example, Greenfield, Kaplan, and Ware, 1985). Often, however, these programs are implemented and evaluated without an explicit, overarching framework or model for chronic illness management.

To complete this picture, pharmaceutical companies have recently asserted their strong interest in developing chronic illness management models (Cunningham, 1997). They have this interest because medication management plays such a vital role in the treatment of some chronic illnesses (Zalta, Eichner, and Henry, 1994). Many pharmaceutical companies now offer managed care organizations and large, self-insured employers services that "range from patient and provider education to practice guidelines and outcomes measurement" (Taylor, 1995, p. 11). The goal is to reduce hospitalizations and emergency room use while improving quality through enhanced medication management. Some providers have expressed skepticism about these initiatives, however, viewing them primarily as vehicles for increasing pharmaceutical sales (Taylor, 1995, p. 13).

Clearly, there are clinical, economic, and entrepreneurial pressures for change in the organization, delivery, and financing of care for persons with chronic illnesses. At this point, it is entirely uncertain what the ultimate outcome will be as these pressures converge. They underscore the urgent need to assess what is known and what is reasonable in the treatment of chronic illnesses. These pressures also highlight the importance of developing a framework and set of principles for chronic illness management that can be implemented and sustained in real-world settings.

2

Defining the Chronic Illness Management Team

The treatment of chronic illnesses is usually thought to consist of distinct but interconnected activities. The first set of activities relates to identifying the illness. Typically, this is accomplished through diagnostic tests, investigation into the patient's history, and clinical observation of the patient.

Once the illness has been diagnosed with a reasonable level of certainty, agreement must be reached about a treatment plan. In addition to incorporating what is clinically known about the illness's responsiveness to medications, physical therapy, and other interventions, treatment plans must accommodate patient preferences and reflect the availability and accessibility of treatment resources.

Once a treatment plan has been established, the focus shifts to implementation. Successful implementation occurs when the plan's various elements (for example, the taking of medications) are carried out over a period of time. Implementing the plan well could also mean adjusting it if resource availability or patient preferences change.

The final activity in the treatment of chronic illnesses involves monitoring the impact of treatment on the patient. With respect to chronic illnesses, this means tracking change in a patient's physical, social, and psychological functioning.

Traditional Caregiver Roles

Altogether, the activities associated with treating a chronic illness typically involve a large number of individuals and organizations. The roles they play in the treatment process vary with the type of chronic illness, patient and family characteristics, and clinician training and preferences, among other factors.

Defining the Patient's Role

One of the fundamental characteristics of chronic illness is that a cure, in the traditional sense, is not expected. This means that the patient must accommodate the limitations that the illness imposes on everyday life, with a high likelihood of deterioration in function over time (Corbin and Strauss, 1987). In reality, "chronically ill people suffer from leading restricted lives, experiencing a sense of social isolation, being discredited, and burdening others" (Conrad, 1987, p. 12). This can strain relationships with family members on whom the patient relies for help in treating and coping with the illness. The limitations imposed by the illness can be unpredictable on a day-to-day basis. In the absence of a physician or other trained health professional, the patient must frequently adjust medication levels and physical activity and monitor functioning. As Wiener (1975) observes with respect to arthritis patients, "On any given day they do not know beforehand about symptoms: (1) presence (if there will be any pain, swelling, or stiffness), (2) place (area of bodily involvement), (3) quantity (degree of disabling intensity), or (4) temporality (whether onset will be gradual or sudden), as well as duration and frequency of flare-ups" (quoted in Conrad, 1987, p. 8). Patient management of symptoms is complicated by the side effects that accompany many of the medications used to treat chronic illnesses. Consequently, patient evaluation of the trade-off between side effects and symptom relief becomes an important consideration in the management of chronic illness. Medical professionals cannot evaluate this factor without direct patient input.

These considerations support the idea of emphasizing patient education in the management of many chronic illnesses, such as asthma, diabetes, and hypertension (McCann and Blossom, 1990). The medical professional is seen as the educator and the patient as the student. The patient learns about the nature of the disease, its typical course, the type of interventions (often pharmaceutical) that can alter this course or alleviate symptoms, and—most important— the responsibility that the patient has for implementing these interventions (Ammerman and others, 1992). In effect, the patient is enlisted as a participant in his or her own treatment, with expectations and responsibilities clearly defined (Speedling and Rose, 1985; Haynes, Wang, and Gomes, 1987; Garrity, 1981; Mulley, Mendoza, Rockefeller, and Staker, 1996; Wise, 1993).

This approach raises several obvious questions about the management of the illness. For example, What are the limits of the patient's responsibilities? Who should play the educator role? When should the patient be the educator and the caregiver the student? How can the patient be motivated to manage the illness effectively? The answers to these questions and, ultimately, the definition of the patient's role will vary with patient and disease characteristics and with providers' willingness to engage the patient fully in managing the illness (Haug and Lavin, 1981).

Recognizing the Demands on Primary Care Physicians

The Institute of Medicine (IOM) defines primary care as "the provision of integrated, accessible health services by clinicians who are accountable for addressing a large majority of personal health care needs, developing a sustained partnership with patients, and practicing in the context of family and community" (Institute of Medicine, 1994). This definition emphasizes the process of providing primary care rather than any particular person. Another definition of a primary care physician says that someone with that title has training, practices medicine, and receives continuing medical education in "health promotion and disease prevention, assessment and evaluation of common symptoms and physical signs, management of common acute and chronic medical conditions, [and] identification and appropriate referral for other needed medical services" (Council on Graduate Medical Education, 1992). By these definitions, the primary care physician is expected to play a significant role in the management of chronic illness.

There are several logical reasons for the primary care physician to play a leadership role in treating chronic illness (Williams, 1994). First, the primary care physician will likely be the first medical professional to have contact with the patient concerning the illness and will also likely play an important part in reaching an initial diagnosis and prescribing treatment (Schellevis and others, 1993). Second, by virtue of his or her training, experience, and position within the medical care delivery system, the primary care physician is well positioned to play a linking role, interacting with specialists, case managers, hospital staff, family members, and others who might be involved in the delivery of care (Dietrich and others, 1988). Third, this leadership role is typically ratified by health care purchasers, who view primary care physicians as less costly than specialists. If a primary care physician plays a leadership role, health care purchasers also see that as more cost effective than uncoordinated care characterized by "doctor shopping" and uninformed use of medications.

Although there clearly is a need for the primary care physician to be involved, a leadership role for this physician may not always be appropriate in the management of chronic illness. Primary care physicians, especially within evolving managed care systems, have great demands placed on their time in the course of normal practice. An ongoing leadership role in coordinating and managing treatment for an individual with a chronic illness, possibly characterized by complicated comorbid conditions, simply may not be an efficient use of primary care physician time. Also, when the patient's condition is severe, the primary care physician may not possess the specialized clinical knowledge necessary to coordinate treatment effectively (Newton, Hayes, and Hutchinson, 1991). For these reasons, it seems likely that the primary care physician's appropriate role in managing chronic illness will vary with the illness's nature, progression, and the availability and competence of other possible participants in the care management process.

Taking Advantage of Specialized Knowledge

In theory, because primary care is an activity, the same physician could provide primary care to some patients and more specialized services to others. In practice, this seems to be the case for many internal medicine subspecialists. Almost twenty years ago, Aiken and others (1979) found that cardiologists, rheumatologists, endocrinologists, pulmonologists, gastroenterologists, and allergists were heavily involved in the delivery of primary care and that about 20 percent of patients received their primary care from subspecialists.

Subspecialists' provision of primary care is arguably most appropriate, and most common in practice, for patients with chronic health problems in the subspecialist's area of expertise (Westbom and Kornfält, 1991). To formalize this notion, the American Society of Internal Medicine cites the concept of *principal care*, which it defines as "integrated, accessible health care provided by medical subspecialists and neurologists that addresses the large majority of the personal health care needs of patients with chronic conditions requiring the subspecialist's expertise, and for whom the subspecialist assumes care management, developing a sustained physician-patient partnership and practicing within the context of family and community" (1995, p. 10). There is no doubt that, by this definition, specialists could play a leadership role in the management of chronic illness. (See Mendenhall, Moynihan, and Radecki, 1984, for an analysis of the principal care approach.)

At a minimum, because specialists are likely to have more knowledge about a particular chronic condition than any other individual involved in its treatment, they can exert a powerful influence on the allocation of treatment resources and responsibilities. Purchasers of care, including managed care organizations, frequently express concern over how specialists' involvement will increase treatment costs (Kassirer, 1994). Specialty-dominated care is often perceived to be expensive and oriented toward a "medical model" of treatment. In addition to its cost, a potential drawback of this medical model is that it may not give enough weight to the nonmedical services needed to manage chronic illnesses or to the importance of the patient and the patient's family in illness management (Braunwald, 1991). Therefore, although specialists contribute valuable disease-specific expertise to the treatment of chronic illness, it may not be appropriate for them to assume leadership roles in the overall management of care. As with the primary care physician, however, this is likely to depend on such factors as the stage of the illness, the need for the specialist's expertise in its ongoing management, and the training and practice styles of individual specialists.

Expanding the Responsibilities of Nonphysicians

Some experts believe that the effective management of chronic illnesses requires ongoing and relatively frequent contact between the patient and a health professional trained specifically in the treatment of the illness. It does not necessarily follow, however, that a physician must be in this role (Pigg, 1988). For both financial and clinical reasons, it may be more appropriate for a nurse, nurse practitioner, or other health professional to maintain contact with the patient and the patient's family (Campbell, Mauksch, Neikirk, and Hosokawa, 1990), enlisting the physician's help as needed. This health professional is typically responsible for ongoing patient and family education and might play a case management or coordination role, linking the patient and family with community services and support groups as necessary (White, Gundrum, Shearer, and Simmons, 1994).

Because the nonphysician health professional theoretically plays this mediating function and is an important source of information about the illness, he or she has a potentially powerful position. The health professional influences information flows relating to care management and, possibly, the patient's access to the specialist's expertise. Despite the importance of this role, in most organizational settings the nonphysician health professional is not regarded as the leader of the care process. In providing overall direction for treatment, this person usually defers to the physician's judgment. Also, there may not be clear sources of reimbursement for all of the health professional's efforts, creating a discord between theory and practice as it relates to the nonphysician health professional's role in managing chronic illnesses.

Supporting the Activities of the Patient's Family

The family's potential importance in managing the chronic illness is widely acknowledged. According to Conrad (1987), "There can be little doubt that families are pivotal actors in the world of illness. Families are important as interpreters, caretakers, support systems, and buffers; chronic illness also can place different strains and new burdens on family life" (p. 15). In the literature on chronic illness, the family's role is discussed most frequently as it relates to illnesses affecting children, such as pediatric asthma. In these cases, Bishop, Woll, and Arango (1993) observe that "with their knowledge regarding certain aspects of a child's condition, professionals at times may lose sight of the fact that the family is the center and the constant in the child's world, whereas professionals move in and out. . . . The family is intimately familiar with the strengths and abilities of the child, the challenges of providing care and the needs of others in the family. This knowledge is critical to the success of any health care plan" (quoted in Ahmann, 1994, p. 114).

Taking a more general perspective, Strauss, Fagerhaugh, Suczek, and Wiener (1985) have introduced the notion of "kin work" to encompass all of the activities in which family members engage to care for and support chronically ill family members. These activities include help with taking medicine; provision of emotional support; and assistance with driving, cooking, bathing, managing financial affairs, and so forth. As with patients, family members are frequently enlisted by medical care providers in educational programs (Morisky and others, 1985) and in support groups designed to facilitate the overall management of the chronic illness (Marcenko and Smith, 1992). The family's role is circumscribed by factors such as the illness's nature and progression, the family's emotional and financial resources, and the frequently observed unwillingness of those with chronic diseases to "burden" family members.

Linking with the Social Service System

The consequences of lived-with chronic illnesses tend to be social, as well as medical (Schlesinger, 1986; Schlesinger and Mechanic, 1993). Persons with chronic illnesses are often restricted in their abilities to meet their responsibilities at work and to maintain normal relations with family and friends. Because of the long-term nature of chronic illnesses, these restrictions are not temporary and, in fact, may worsen over time. Therefore, an important part of managing chronic illness is providing or coordinating services that enhance the patient's ability to lead as normal a life as possible.

Depending on the nature and severity of the illness, these services could include personal care, transportation, or help with housework, chores, shopping, and similar daily activities. The providers of these services constitute the social service system at the community level. The interface of social and medical services in the treatment of chronic diseases has been controversial. Social service providers are concerned that clinicians are not sufficiently knowledgeable about their capabilities or appreciative of their potential to contribute to the ongoing management of chronic illnesses. Medical service providers have difficulty assessing the need for, and the effectiveness of, many social services, and they often find the quality of social services to vary greatly.

Special Problems in Managing Chronic Illnesses

Our discussion of treating chronic illnesses has thus far focused on clinical characteristics that distinguish these illnesses from other medical conditions, as well as on the individuals and organizations that have historically been involved in their treatment. The discussion has touched on at least four specific considerations with particular implications for chronic illness management.

• Chronic illnesses are fundamentally longitudinal in nature. To be successful, a chronic illness management model will need to be sustainable over time and flexible enough to adjust to changes in the patient's condition and the environment in which treatment takes place (Corbin and Strauss, 1991; Walker, 1991).

• The treatment of chronic illnesses requires a greater breadth of resources and a larger number of individuals than the treatment of most acute problems. In adapting to their illnesses, patients often require social as well as medical services. Even within the medical sphere, many different types of treatment resources may be used, because chronic illnesses are frequently accompanied by other medical problems. Clearly, the effective coordination of services is critical to the success of any chronic illness management model (Starfield, Simborg, Horn, and Yourtee, 1976).

• The patient and the family are likely to be involved, in a very central way, in the treatment of chronic illness. This raises several questions that need to be addressed in the design of a chronic illness management model: How will treatment goals be determined? How can patients and family members work most effectively with medical and social service providers in treating illnesses? How can family members sustain their participation in the treatment process over time?

• It is difficult to measure success in the treatment of chronic illnesses. In the short run, there may be clear indicators of successful symptom control (for example, peak-flow meter readings for asthma). In the longer term, however, a downward trajectory of patient functioning is characteristic of many chronic illnesses (Gillick, 1984). Some analysts argue that traditional physiological measures of functioning are defined too narrowly to provide an adequate picture of treatment effectiveness. They also believe that this bigger picture should include measures of a patient's satisfaction and assessments of the patient's adjustment to the limitations imposed by the illness. A lack of consensus about how to measure the success of treatment presents obstacles to the evaluation of different treatment models and to the provision of effective performance feedback to providers.

A Brief History of Team Care in Chronic Illness Treatment

Given the large number of individuals with varying expertise and perspectives who are likely to be involved in treating people with chronic illnesses, there is a clear need to coordinate their efforts. One coordinating mechanism that has received some attention in the health care literature is the concept of the health care team.

Traditionally, the treatment of illness has been portrayed as a series of physician-patient interactions in which the physician's technical expertise is used in diagnosing the problem, selecting an intervention, and implementing treatment. The patient's role in this interaction is to follow the physician's instructions so that a cure might be obtained as expeditiously as possible (Emanuel and Emanuel, 1992; Brody, 1980). Other health care and social service professionals, including other physicians, are incorporated into the treatment process on an individual basis as their skills are required.

In contrast to this picture of the treatment process, a long-standing literature addresses team processes for health care delivery. Medical historians see the development of the treatment team concept in U.S. medicine as consisting of three distinct periods (Brown, 1982). First, before World War II, there was recognition that the practice of medicine was becoming more science-based and more complicated and that new approaches would be needed to integrate specialized knowledge into the treatment process systematically.

Then, after World War II, these prewar trends continued, as evidenced by a dramatic increase in the number of new specialties and of new technologies. The need for "comprehensive care" was widely recognized, as was the need to involve health professionals and social service providers at all levels of care (Keith, 1991). One response, at the conceptual level, was to develop the "health team" model. *Team care* was defined as "coordinated, comprehensive care provided by persons who integrate their observations, expertise and decisions" (Halstead, 1976). This model had broad appeal as a way of "bringing together the opinions and approaches of specialists to bear upon a problem that cuts across their specialties" (Nagi, 1975). Plus, this model was expected to facilitate collaboration between primary care physicians and specialists, use nonphysician personnel effectively in the treatment process, and include patients more systematically in treating their own illnesses.

Although a great deal of literature in the 1960s and early 1970s praised the potential of the health team model, two comprehensive literature reviews published in the mid-1970s found relatively little empirical support for the presumed benefits of team care. Nagi (1975, p. 87) concluded that "the vast majority of the literature on teamwork is descriptive and prescriptive rather than analytical. Data are generated from case studies with little theoretical orientation."

Halstead (1976) reached a similar conclusion in his review of the literature on team care in treating chronic illness. He found that "over a twenty-five-year period, an avalanche of articles and reports has been published which almost unanimously endorse the proposition that team care is desirable, relevant and effective in many areas of health cure delivery. Yet the evidence to support these claims is exceedingly slim" (pp. 509–510). In his view, this literature "helped create a false sense of legitimacy and effectiveness unwarranted by the facts" (p. 510). To remedy this situation, he recommended that there be carefully structured studies of team models of chronic illness treatment. These studies would focus on a homogeneous diagnostic category; include random assignment with a comparison group representing standard treatment; and collect both process and outcome data, including patient psychosocial-functional status and long-term follow-up information.

Since the 1970s, a large number of studies have attempted to provide an empirical basis for the development of team care approaches for the treatment of chronic illness. The findings from many of those studies will be summarized in the next chapter.

3

Learning from Clinical Research

This chapter summarizes selected findings from the clinical literature that relate to chronic illness treatment models. Space limitations make it impossible to include detailed descriptions of individual studies or findings from all relevant studies. The discussion is organized according to five chronic illnesses that are relatively common in general practice: asthma, arthritis, diabetes, hypertension, and stable coronary artery disease. In each case, issues relative to patient education and the use of treatment teams are discussed because of the frequency with which they are incorporated in chronic illness treatment models. The concluding section draws some general lessons from this research.

Asthma

Asthma affects more than 5 percent of the U.S. population at an estimated annual cost of $6.2 billion (Zablocki, 1995; Evans and others, 1987; Weiss, Gergen, and Hodgson, 1992). According to the Centers for Disease Control (1995), emergency visits and hospitalizations accounted for 60 percent of total costs. Among children, asthma is the most common chronic medical condition and accounts for more absenteeism from school, emergency room visits, and hospitalizations than any other childhood condition (Hughes, McLeod, Garner, and Goldbloom, 1991).

These estimates of disease prevalence and economic impact are among the reasons that asthma has been identified as a prototypical disease for a chronic illness management model (Kretz and Meyer, 1993). Another impetus for developing asthma management programs is that inpatient admission rates for asthma are one of the measures of health care quality, according to the Health Plans Employer Data and Information Set, which has been developed to compare health maintenance organizations (Zablocki, 1995). Therefore, reducing asthma inpatient admissions is important to health plans hoping to increase their standing with employers. The potential for patient self-management and the ability to quantify outcomes have led some to estimate that a potential cost savings of 25 percent can be achieved through appropriate management of asthma (Todd, 1995).

Patient Education

Educating patients about how they can manage their asthma has demonstrated effectiveness and cost savings in a number of studies (Mayo, Richman, and Harris, 1990; Wilson and others, 1993; Charlton, Charlton, Broomfield, and Mullee, 1991; Charlton, Charlton, Broomfield, and Campbell, 1992). Given the proven effectiveness of patient education, it is not surprising that many models for asthma management include an educational component.

For example, one study of ambulatory patients enrolled in a staff-model HMO found that instructing children and their families in asthma management, medications, asthma triggers, and use of inhalers and peak-flow meters decreased emergency room visit rates by 79 percent and hospital admissions by 86 percent (Greineder, Loane, and Parks, 1995). Similarly, a randomized study found that a medical treatment and education program reduced hospital readmissions threefold and hospital days twofold (Mayo, Richman, and Harris, 1990). Instruction in asthma self-management at a nurse-run asthma clinic led to a reduction in patient morbidity and a decrease in physician workload (Charlton, Charlton, Broomfield, and Mullee, 1991). The latter study also found that patient self-education alleviated feelings of stigma and increased patient confidence in the efficacy of the care provided by both the patient and the physician (Charlton, Charlton, Broomfield, and Campbell, 1992). Finally, a review of self-management initiatives for children suggests that these programs can reduce the number of emergency room and unscheduled physician visits, as well as improve patient participation in physical and social activities (Boner and Valletta, 1994).

Lewis and others (1984) found that, for children between the ages of eight and twelve, an education program's costs were offset by savings from fewer emergency room visits and days of hospitalization. These reductions in service use generated an estimated savings of $180 per child per year for those who received the educational program, compared with a control group. In contrast, however, Bailey and colleagues (1990) found that while patient education increased adherence to treatment regimens and functional status for asthma patients, program costs outweighed savings.

The person who administers self-management clinics or sessions for patients is typically a nurse (Hughes, McLeod, Garner, and Goldbloom, 1991; Wilson and others, 1993; Charlton, Charlton, Broomfield, and Mullee, 1991; Charlton, Charlton, Broomfield, and Campbell, 1992) or in some cases a health education specialist (Windsor and others, 1990; Bailey and others, 1990). Health education experts develop educational materials, which physicians then review. Despite the widespread acceptance of the need to involve patients with chronic illness in their own care, Boner and Valleta (1994) caution that complete patient self-management may be an inappropriate goal, because it implies that patients treat themselves without physician guidance. Instead, management programs should foster a "partnership" or "cooperative management" relationship between physicians, patients, and families.

Role of Primary Care and Specialist Physicians

An important issue in asthma management concerns the roles of specialists and primary care physicians. One recent study compared referral patterns of pediatricians and general practitioners for asthma, congenital heart disease, and diabetes (Blancquaert, Zvagulis, Gray-Donald, and Pless, 1992). In general, pediatricians referred their patients to specialists less often than general practitioners did, and patterns of referral depended primarily on clinical condition. Pediatricians referred about 26 percent of their asthma patients, compared with 46 percent for general practitioners.

Some research suggests that asthma patients under specialists' care are treated more aggressively than primary care physicians' patients. For example, Engel, Freund, Stein, and Fletcher (1989) found that allergists treated patients more intensively than primary care physicians, as measured by the proportion of patients receiving oral corticosteroids in the study period; this difference could not be explained by patient selection or severity of condition. Freund and others (1989) reported a higher cost of care per patient for allergists, primarily because of the use of more expensive medications.

A case can be made, however, that specialists' treatment of appropriate asthma patients may be more cost effective than their treatment by primary care physicians (Todd, 1995). Zieger and others (1991) compared asthma care delivered by allergists and generalist physicians. In their study, patients treated by an allergist experienced a 50 percent reduction in emergency room visits and made greater use of inhaled corticosteroids and cromolyn, compared with patients treated by generalist physicians.

An innovative asthma treatment program in Scotland addressed the issue of coordination of asthma care among physicians (van Damme, Drummond, Beattie, and Douglas, 1994). Asthma patients who were sixteen or older made annual visits to a hospital-based specialist but remained in close contact with their general practitioner, who gave the specialist updates via a computerized patient record system. In this program, general practitioners had a distinct primary care role and viewed the specialist providers as troubleshooters and educators. Communication between physicians and patients was coordinated by a computerized patient record system that generated letters to patients every three months inviting them to consult with their general practitioner. Patients also received a questionnaire about their condition, with the responses entered into the computerized patient record.

Treatment Teams

Several different program designs that rely on treatment teams have been proposed for asthma treatment. Some have been tested, and others have not. For example, the Denver-based National Jewish Center for Immunology and Respiratory Medicine has developed a program called Time Out for Asthma. The program was designed for patients of all ages with severe asthma, although patients with less severe conditions can also take part (Mason, Katz, and Bethel, 1994; Rohl, Meyer, and Lung, 1994; Todd, 1995). Patients treated under this model have typically had multiple hospitalizations or emergency room visits before entering the program and have thereby incurred substantial medical costs. The program entails intensive, one-week, outpatient treatment. During this time, a multidisciplinary team works with patients and family members to develop individualized, comprehensive treatment plans. Registered nurses with respiratory training act as "case managers" for the patients (Rohl, Meyer, and Lung, 1994). The team also seeks to determine if a patient's asthma attacks are triggered by environmental factors. The patient's treatment plan is discussed with the referring physician, and patients learn self-management skills so that they can more effectively control their conditions and prevent acute asthmatic episodes (Rohl, Meyer, and Lung, 1994).

Kaiser Permanente has implemented a program for pediatric asthma patients that includes patient and family education on a variety of factors, such as the use of peak-flow measurements, spacers for metered dose inhalers, use of compressor-driven nebulizers, and early use of steroids during asthma flare-ups (Zablocki, 1995; Stevens and Weiss-Harrison, 1993). For pediatricians, the program emphasizes that asthma attacks can be prevented through medication and that hospitalizations and emergency room visits represent "failures." For patients, a respiratory therapist provides home instruction on the use of a peak-flow meter and nebulizer, with the health plan covering the costs of this instruction. Physicians at Kaiser credit the new asthma management approach with a decrease in the number of hospital days and hospital admissions (Zablocki, 1995).

Miller and Wood (1991) highlight the need for personalized treatment programs in their description of a conceptual model of childhood asthma care. They propose a comprehensive, multidisciplinary approach that involves the child, family, school administrators, teachers, and peers. Their model emphasizes developmental issues that are specific to a pediatric population. Experts at the National Jewish Center for Immunology and Respiratory Medicine estimate that between 70 to 95 percent of pediatric and adolescent asthma patients have psychosocial problems that interfere with their course of treatment (Todd, 1995). They estimate that 30 to 50 percent of severe asthmatics in the general population have some level of psychosocial problems that affect their treatment.

Conclusions

One summary of the literature on asthma management (Todd, 1995) suggests that case management is the key to a successful program but is not always fully integrated into programs. The lack of consistency in managing asthma demonstrates the need for a systematic method of evaluating both patient and physician. Todd also draws the following conclusions:

- Not enough emphasis is placed on psychosocial issues.

- Patient education is imperative, but current methods may not be effective.

- The role of specialist physicians in ongoing treatment can be reduced.

- There is a lack of data on the costs and benefits of current management models.

- Outcomes measurements are typically limited to utilization review, hospitalizations, and emergency room visits, and these measurements are entirely absent in many early intervention efforts.

- Implementing measurement systems is difficult but important.

- For patients with severe asthma, a comprehensive, multidisciplinary treatment program works best.

Although asthma management programs tend to have some of these elements, such as patient education initiatives and a role for case management, other program elements are only partly present because programs were developed to fit the needs of particular patient populations. For example, some programs were developed for severe asthmatics, whereas others were designed for patients with less severe forms of illness. Similarly, some programs were developed specifically for children, whereas others focus on adults. In the same vein, some programs targeted enrollees in a managed care setting, and others were intended for hospital outpatients. Ultimately, it is clear that many of the asthma management programs described in the literature have not been replicated in alternative health care settings or assessed for long-term effects.

Arthritis

The term *arthritis* is commonly used to describe more than one hundred diseases affecting joints and surrounding tissues (Lorig, Konkol, and Gonzalez, 1987), with the most common being osteoarthritis

(Verbrugge and Patrick, 1995). Arthritis affects not only the joints but also the tendons, ligaments, and muscles surrounding joints. It is characterized by pain caused by inflammation, swelling, or joint deformity. In addition to having painful joints, patients with arthritis can experience limited motion, stiffness, fatigue, and depression (Lorig and others, 1994). Arthritis is the most common chronic condition afflicting those who are middle aged and older (Verbrugge and Patrick, 1995); approximately 55 percent of the elderly U.S. population has some form of arthritis, and more than 75 percent of this group is somewhat limited in physical activity (Yelin, 1992). Arthritis results in more work lost than any other chronic condition and, among working-age adults, more people have arthritis in conjunction with other chronic health problems than have arthritis alone (Yelin, 1992). Compared with other chronic conditions, arthritis ranks low in terms of hospital use; the hospitalization rate for patients with arthritis, for example, is one-third of that for patients with diabetes and one-fifth of that for people with heart disease.

Arthritis treatment approaches described in the literature typically have the following goals: to improve physical function; to minimize pain, disability, and deformity; and to diminish the social and psychological dysfunction that can accompany arthritis (Lorig, Konkol, and Gonzalez, 1987). However, the emphasis on specific goals can vary across different forms of the disease. For example, rheumatic diseases in children frequently present special challenges for arthritis management. For this group, specific goals of treatment include preservation of joint function, pain management, and maintenance of self-esteem and self-image (Hughes and D'Ambrosia, 1993).

Patient Education

Self-care and self-management education programs for patients with arthritis are generally viewed as complements to, and not replacements for, professional health care (Lorig, Konkol, and Gonzalez, 1987). Educational programs typically emphasize exercise, relaxation, compliance with treatment regimen, and joint protection (Lorig, Konkol, and Gonzalez, 1987). Lorig, Konkol, and Gonzalez (1987) suggest that, because pain is a primary concern for most patients, pain control should be a major focus of educational programs. Some studies have demonstrated that pain may be reduced by cognitive techniques and possibly through physical exercise.

Self-care activities, such as exercise and joint protection, are thought to be particularly important for patients with rheumatoid arthritis (Neuberger, Smith, Black, and Hassanein, 1993). A recent pilot study assessed the impact of an individualized instructional program for patients with rheumatoid arthritis; the study found that the program improved patient knowledge and adherence to self-care protocols (Neuberger, Smith, Black, and Hassanein, 1993).

A different study compared a home-study model, a small-group model, and a control group in terms of their effects on arthritis self-care. In contrast to the control group, both models were seen to improve patients' arthritis knowledge, self-care, perceived helplessness, and pain (Goeppinger and others, 1989). The small-group intervention had a greater impact on pain and depression, whereas the home care model caused a greater reduction in perceived helplessness.

The Arthritis Self-Management Program (ASMP) developed at Stanford University is intended to improve the behavior, self-efficacy, and health status of patients with arthritis (Lorig and Holman, 1993). With more than fourteen years of development and testing, the ASMP has been disseminated widely in the United States, Canada, and Australia. It is a twelve-hour program, taught at community sites over six weeks by laypersons who, quite frequently, have arthritis themselves. Participants are advised on the uses and effects of medications, exercise, pain management, nutrition, patient-physician communications, and solutions to disease-related problems (Lorig and Holman, 1993). Studies of the ASMP indicate that self-care education has a positive effect on several important patient outcomes and can also reduce costs (Lorig and others, 1985;

Lorig, Mazonson, and Holman, 1993; Lorig and Holman, 1993). One study found that the ASMP reduced pain and decreased costs for both rheumatoid arthritis and osteoarthritis patients compared with a control group (Lorig, Mazonson, and Holman, 1993). The study also found, however, that physical disability increased slightly for the intervention group compared with the control group.

Measuring the success of arthritis programs can be problematic. Because arthritis symptoms can emerge and disappear on a cyclical basis, patients may enter a study during times when they are experiencing symptoms. Patients who are in a control group may seek relief for pain and other symptoms outside of the study; as a result, they may also show improvement. Thus, the tendency for patients to seek care at the bottom of the disease cycle means that patients in both treatment and comparison groups are likely to improve somewhat. This makes it difficult to distinguish the effect of treatment (Lorig, Konkol, and Gonzalez, 1987). Also, in studies examining changes in symptoms over longer time periods, improvement may be unlikely. Because arthritis is a degenerative condition, disability tends to increase over time, although other symptoms may be highly variable. If the measure of disability remains stable, then a finding of no change may be viewed as a positive effect rather than a negative or neutral one (Lorig, Konkol, and Gonzalez, 1987).

A meta-analysis of fifteen studies on how educational interventions affect individuals with rheumatoid arthritis or osteoarthritis indicated that education can improve patient health in a number of areas, including pain, depression, and disability (Mullen, Laville, Biddle, and Lorig, 1987). For rheumatoid arthritis patients, the effects of educational interventions on pain and depression were found to be modest, but these findings were reported as clinically significant, given the nature of the condition.

A new approach to education and self-management, the Patient Partners in Arthritis, was recently initiated as a pilot program by five HMOs (Bilodeau, 1995). Patients currently suffering from arthritis lead the workshops, which both physicians and patients attend. The workshops emphasize self-care, lifestyle changes, and patient empowerment through education about the disease. The workshop leaders also provide specific advice for improving patient-physician relationships through better communication. The project goals are to improve patient self-reliance and satisfaction while decreasing unnecessary office visits and surgeries and avoiding overuse of medications. A formal evaluation of this project has not yet been completed.

Treatment Teams

Providers and ancillary staff on arthritis care teams can include a rheumatologist, nurse, physiotherapist, occupational therapist, physical therapist, social worker, dietitian, podiatrist, psychologist or other mental health specialist, and orthopedic surgeon for patients with an operable condition (Ahlmen, Bjelle, and Sullivan, 1991; Raspe, Deck, and Mattussek, 1992; Schned and others, 1995; Duff, Carpenter, and Neukom, 1974). Team members' roles vary, depending on the specific model, although the primary decision maker for patient care in these models is generally the rheumatologist.

The results from studies evaluating a team care approach to arthritis are mixed. Some studies have found that a team approach is more effective than a nonteam approach in some respects (Ahlmen, Sullivan, and Bjelle, 1988; Duff, Carpenter, and Neukom, 1974), whereas other studies have found no difference in outcomes for experimental and control groups (Schned and others, 1995; Raspe, Deck, and Mattussek, 1992). Several possible explanations have been offered as to why team care approaches to arthritis treatment do not always improve patient outcomes:

- Measurement instruments may be too insensitive to detect small changes.

- The aggregate interventions of the team approach may be too weak to demonstrate substantial changes.

- In some studies, patients and providers know about the intervention, thereby introducing the potential for biases.

- The assumption that a team approach will demonstrate differences in outcomes early in the disease process may be false; longer follow-up periods may be necessary.

- When study patients are well educated with respect to their disease, team approaches with educational components may not represent a significant change from usual care (Schned and others, 1995).

Studies of team care approaches for treatment of juvenile rheumatoid arthritis and other forms of juvenile chronic arthritis are not as prevalent as studies about adults with rheumatoid arthritis. Care and management of arthritis in children may present unique challenges that differ from those for adult patients. For example, children's compliance with prescribed treatment methods is likely to be a greater problem than with adults. One study found that parents of patients with juvenile rheumatoid arthritis reported more compliance with doing range-of-motion exercises and wearing splints than with taking medication (Rapoff, Lindsley, and Christophersen, 1985). Additionally, family may play a larger role in managing a child's arthritis compared with the situation for an adult patient, and counseling may be necessary for families as well as for children (Ansell, 1994).

Conclusions

From a provider perspective, arthritis differs from other chronic illnesses in several ways. For example, physicians may take more time to establish a diagnosis of arthritis than with other conditions (Schned and others, 1995), because a premature or misdiagnosis of arthritis can have serious adverse consequences for a patient. Some specialists believe that the diagnosis of arthritis and development of a care plan are better accomplished by a rheumatologist than a primary care physician and that early referral can be cost effective in the long run (Schned and others, 1995). Indeed, a majority of the arthritis management models involve a specialist as the primary decision maker for patient care. In evaluations of arthritis management programs, success is often difficult to measure (Lynch and Caughey, 1995). A lack of measurable results can be problematic, because a comprehensive team approach can be more costly than traditional care.

Diabetes

Diabetes mellitus is a group of chronic disorders characterized by abnormalities in carbohydrate, protein, and fat metabolism. The common denominator is hyperglycemia, or excess sugar in the blood (Rifkin and Porte, 1990). Prolonged hyperglycemia is a toxic condition that can produce both microvascular and macrovascular damage over time (Walker, 1991). As such, diabetes is a major cause of mortality and morbidity, much of which is preventable (British Multicentre Study Group, 1977; Parving and Hommel, 1989; Bild and others, 1989).

The nearly eight million known cases of diabetes in the United States, together with an estimated eight million undetected cases, represent a prevalence of 6 percent in the United States; this makes diabetes one of the most widespread chronic diseases (Mazze, Bergenstal, and Ginsberg, 1995). Of those individuals with diabetes, about 4 percent have type I (insulin-dependent) diabetes, and the remainder have type II (adult-onset, or non-insulin-dependent) diabetes. As many as 18 percent of people over age sixty-five have type II diabetes (McLemoe and Delozier, 1987). Each year, diabetes is a contributing or underlying cause in approximately 350,000 deaths (American Diabetes Association, 1993). Diabetes is the seventh leading cause of visits to primary care physicians (McLemoe and Delozier, 1987), who spend an average of 8 percent of their time with patients with diabetes (Hiss, 1986).

Despite the finding of the Diabetes Control and Complications Trial (DCCT) that tight glycemic control can prevent or slow the progression of microvascular complications in patients with type I diabetes (Mazze, Bergenstal, and Ginsberg, 1995), as few as 15 percent of adults with diabetes achieve normal levels of glycosylated hemoglobin, or hemoglobin A_1C (HbA_{1C}), and even worse results have been observed in children (Mann and Johnston, 1982; Gonen and Horwitz, 1977; Tattersall and McMulloch, 1984).

Role of Primary Care and Specialist Physicians

Traditionally, either the primary care physician or the diabetes specialist (diabetologist, endocrinologist) has been the chief (and frequently sole) caregiver and decision maker in the treatment of diabetes patients. However, the primary care physician often has limited time to spend with any one patient and must respond to multiple complaints during this time. Consequently, because of its complicated nature, the quality of care for diabetes may suffer. Indeed, Hayes and Harries (1984) found in a randomized controlled trial in the United Kingdom that fewer patients cared for in general practice (where they were seen by a primary care physician) were reviewed regularly or had their blood glucose concentration tested regularly, as compared with patients seen primarily in a hospital diabetic clinic (treated by a diabetes specialist). Also, more patients in the general practice group than those in the hospital clinic were admitted to the hospital, and more of the general practice patients died during the study. Finally, the mean concentrations of HbA_{1C} were higher in the general practice group patients.

The provision of routine care by a diabetes specialist can be costly and, because the specialist sees the patient only for diabetes, it can also be fragmented; the diabetologist sets insulin schedules, the cardiologist prescribes medication for hypertension and dyslipidemia, and so forth. Comorbid conditions and pregnancies increase the importance of coordinating care among multiple specialists and the primary care physician.

Treatment Teams

Some authors stress the potential for an enhanced role for the diabetes specialist nurse, who can provide more intensive counseling to patients with diabetes. In the United Kingdom, Siddons and McAughey (1992) promote the development of diabetes specialist nurses through advanced educational programs. The nurse specialist is seen as playing both clinical and consultative roles. Day, Metcalfe, and Johnson (1992), also in the United Kingdom, see the diabetes specialist nurse as a full partner in diabetes care, working in parallel with the primary care physician.

Etzwiler (1972) stresses that, although the physician must be seen as the leader of the medical team, it is crucial that the patient be viewed as its most important member. He feels that educating the patient and accepting the patient as a member of the medical team can reduce costs and improve the quality of health care. In the DCCT, patients were encouraged to assume increased responsibility for their own care and were taught to adjust insulin doses to changes in diet, eating time, activity, stress, and illness. Etzwiler (1972) also emphasizes the importance of the entire family's becoming involved in diabetes care. This is especially important for meal preparation, support for behavioral changes, and compliance with treatment regimens.

A nutritionist also can play a key role in diabetes management (Lyon and Vinci, 1993; Gewirtz, 1994; Koperski, 1992; Kronsbein and others, 1988; Drash, 1994; Siddons and McAughey, 1992). In some models, however, nutrition and diet information is provided by certified diabetes educators (Comi, 1991), physician assistants (Kronsbein and others, 1988), or specially trained nurses (Rosenqvist, Carlson, and Luft, 1988). The treatment team also may include an ophthalmologist, podiatrist, psychologist, and social worker; these professionals may treat patients referred to them as necessary, or they may serve primarily as consultants to the primary care physician.

In developing models of team care, organizational support and staff involvement in decision making are important. Carlson and Rosenqvist (1988) compared clinics that had successfully implemented a diabetes control program with those that had not; these researchers found that successful implementation required staff involvement in the planning process and organization of the routines needed to implement the diabetes program.

Patient Education

Because a patient's lifestyle, compliance with often complicated treatment regimens, and glycemic control all affect the patient's management of the diabetes, patient education has a primary role in models for diabetes care. One study (McDonald, 1968) found that although 77 percent of all patients with diabetes were on some dietary management program, only about 10 percent had a good comprehension of what this involved. In another study, some 150 nurses, dietitians, and physicians surveyed felt that the primary difficulty in treating diabetes patients was "lack of patient knowledge and cooperation" (Etzwiler, 1972).

Almost all diabetes management models recognize this problem and incorporate patient education components. For example, Gibbons and Saunders (1988) describe a protocol in which the nurse provides patient education. Gewirtz (1994) discusses implementing the principles of the DCCT on a broad scale, identifying the nurse educator as the team member who has the greatest personal contact with the patient. Drash (1994) describes a computer-based teaching program for patients with type I diabetes and their families. Kronsbein and others (1988) propose and evaluate a structured teaching program for elderly patients with type II diabetes. Funnell and others (1991) develop the concept of patient empowerment in diabetes care and treatment. They see empowerment as offering a practical, conceptual framework for diabetes patient education by providing the patient with the knowledge, skill, and responsibility to effect change. Empowerment, in their view, can promote overall health and maximize the use of available resources.

Evidence of Effectiveness

Do coordinated models of care improve the care of diabetic patients? Several studies have examined this question. Boucher and others (1987) compared the care of patients in a pilot program (DSS) in an inner-city London district with the care of a similar group receiving usual care at a diabetic clinic (DC). Under the pilot program, the primary care physician was identified as the "responsible doctor." A computer was used to record administrative and clinical data. Computer-generated lists were used to request HbA_{1C} tests on patients and to refer patients to podiatric, dietetic, or ophthalmologic departments. Patients with high HbA_{1C} levels were to be contacted by the responsible doctor. A consultant ophthalmologist trained all primary care physicians in the examination of diabetic fundi. Regular seminars on managing diabetes were held for all primary care physicians and nurses. The DSS patients were seen more often than the DC patients and experienced significant reduction in their HbA_{1C} levels, whereas the DC patients' HbA_{1C} levels remained unchanged.

Koperski (1992) investigated the impact of introducing a method of systematic care into a general practice in inner-city London. The idea was that a "diabetic day" would occur once each month. On the diabetic day, the practice as a whole (especially the practice nurse) saw patients with diabetes. There was a significant improvement in all process measures after introduction of the diabetic day, and there were significant decreases in HbA_{1C} levels after two years. Koperski concluded that the introduction of systematic care into a practice that is already well staffed, organized, and motivated can significantly improve care for diabetic patients.

A similar study (Day, Metcalfe, and Johnson, 1992), also in the United Kingdom, evaluated the effects of an integrated system of diabetes care with an enhanced role for the diabetes specialist nurse. These nurses were established as full counselors in diabetes care. Working with the doctor, the nurses reviewed all patients whose needs were not predominantly medical. The study found significant and sustained falls in HbA_{1C} for the patients whom the nurses saw. There were smaller, but also significant, changes for the patients who continued to attend the routine clinic. Yearly admission rates for ketoacidosis and hypoglycemia fell substantially in the nurse group.

A German study (Kronsbein and others, 1988) evaluated the effects of a structured treatment and teaching program on 114 elderly patients with type II diabetes. The teaching program consisted of teaching sessions of 90 to 120 minutes each week for four weeks. The groups of four to six patients were taught primarily by physician's assistants. After one year, the investigators concluded that the structured treatment and teaching program improved the overall quality of patient care in a general practice setting for non-insulin-dependent diabetic patients.

Because of possible cultural differences, and differences in health care reimbursement systems in Europe and the United States, some aspects of these studies may have limited applicability in this country. For these reasons, two U.S. studies are of particular interest. One, by Mazze and others (1994), applied the type of intensive treatment regimen used in the DCCT to individuals with either type I or type II diabetes in routine practice under the auspices of primary care physicians. The study targeted blood glucose control and used protocols developed by an interdisciplinary team of endocrinologists, perinatologists, family physicians, clinical epidemiologists, nurse clinician specialists in diabetes, dietitians, and psychologists. Patients under this system had more clinic visits and lower HbA_{1C} levels over a six-month period. In contrast, nonprogram patients maintained the same level of glycemia over the study period.

A second U.S. study (Weinberger and others, 1995) evaluated the impact of an intervention on glycemic control and quality-of-life measures (SF-36 scores) for patients with type II diabetes. In this randomized, controlled study, nurses in a primary care setting called patients at least monthly. The nurses reviewed prescribed regimens and significant signs and symptoms of hypoglycemia and hyperglycemia, reinforced the importance of compliance, identified barriers to compliance, and initiated actions to facilitate compliance (for example, alerting physicians and preparing referrals to diet or smoking cessation clinics). After one year, control was significantly better in the intervention group, and fewer diabetes-related signs and symptoms were reported for those patients, but there were no differences in quality-of-life scores.

Conclusions

Based on this literature review, the most important components of a coordinated, potentially cost-effective model for diabetes care appear to be the following:

- An organizational structure and culture that promote the coordination of care between the primary care physician, specialists, and other personnel (nutritionist or dietitian, podiatrist, and psychologist or social worker)

- Treatment based in a primary care setting with support from specialists

- A registry of patients with diabetes to facilitate regular reviews and monitor patients' progress

- A significant role for the nurse-educator or case manager, both to help coordinate care and to educate, counsel, and remind the patient at a level not possible for the primary care physician

- A clearly delineated protocol or guideline for diabetes management

- A recognition of the patient as a key member of the medical team with major responsibilities for both identifying problems and helping to solve them

- Enlistment of the entire family to support behavioral and dietary changes and to be involved in the educational process

Whether such a model can be implemented successfully within existing reimbursement constraints remains an important issue, however—one that existing research has not effectively addressed.

Hypertension

Hypertension, or high blood pressure, is generally defined as a mean systolic blood pressure (SBP) greater than 140 mm Hg or a mean diastolic blood pressure (DBP) greater than 90 mm Hg. Patients are also considered to have hypertension if they are currently being treated for this condition with a prescription medication (Burt and others, 1995). For elderly patients, an elevated SBP can represent a more serious health risk than an elevated DBP (Applegate, 1993). Most providers focus on DBP, however, because it is more highly correlated with organ damage (Applegate, 1993). Hypertension most frequently damages the heart, brain, kidneys, and blood vessels (Savage, McGee, and Oster, 1987).

High blood pressure has been described as one of the most important modifiable risk factors for cardiovascular disease (Burt and others, 1995). People with uncontrolled hypertension are three to four times more likely to develop coronary heart disease than those with normal blood pressure, and those with hypertension are seven times more likely to have a stroke (Healthy People 2000, 1991). Furthermore, hypertension has been identified as the most common risk factor for congestive heart failure (Levy and others, 1996), and it is a common risk factor for myocardial infarction, end-stage renal disease, and peripheral vascular disease (Burt and others, 1995).

Hypertension is the most frequent reason for adult patients to incur outpatient visits, and it accounts for the highest use of prescription drugs in the United States (Harris, Luft, Rudy, and Tierney, 1995). Approximately 30 percent of adults in the U.S. population have high blood pressure (Healthy People 2000, 1991), with its prevalence varying by age, gender, race, income, and geographic region (National Center for Health Statistics, 1994).

Among males younger than age forty-five, the estimated prevalence of hypertension was 3.2 percent in 1994. For men between the ages of forty-five and sixty-four, prevalence soars to 22 percent. It rises to 32 percent for men who are sixty-five and older. Hypertension is considerably more prevalent among African Americans. As income increases, hypertension appears less prevalent. It also appears less prevalent in the West compared with other regions of the country, and it is slightly less prevalent in cities than in nonmetropolitan areas (National Center for Health Statistics, 1994).

The primary treatment goal for hypertension patients is to lower blood pressure and the concomitant risk of complications from cardiovascular disease through the least intrusive means (Whelton and Brancati, 1993). A 1996 report by the World Health Organization recommends that, at the population level, hypertension control should incorporate aspects of primary prevention, early detection, and adequate treatment to prevent complications associated with hypertension (Chalmers and Zanchetti, 1996). At the patient level, this goal can be achieved through a combination of lifestyle modifications, drug therapies, and patient education.

As a first step, providers must select patients who would be most likely to benefit from antihypertensive treatment. Ideally, that would mean those who are most likely to develop clinically manifest disease (MacMahon, 1996). Methods of identifying those patients are not precise, however. Krakoff (1993) found that ambulatory blood pressure monitoring can be used as secondary screening for patients with slightly elevated blood pressure. Costly drug therapy, with side effects that can include sexual dysfunction, can be delayed for 20 to 60 percent of patients who are initially labeled as hypertensive but who, through secondary screening, exhibit lower average daily pressures (Krakoff, 1993). Discontinuation of antihypertensive therapy has been recommended for patients with mild hypertension if they have one or more of the following characteristics: normal body weight, low salt intake, no alcohol consumption, low pretreatment blood pressure, success with one drug only, and no or minimal signs of target organ damage (Schmieder, Rockstroh, and Messerli, 1991).

As antihypertensive drug therapy continues to shift from the use of diuretics and beta-blockers toward the use of more costly calcium channel blockers and ACE inhibitors (Whelton and Brancati, 1993), it becomes increasingly important to assess the cost effectiveness of treatment regimens and to identify patients who would benefit most from treatment. One recommendation is to decide whom to treat based on the patient's total cardiovascular risk, as well as diastolic and systolic blood pressures (Chalmers and Zanchetti, 1996; MacMahon, 1996).

Patient Education

According to Menard and Chatellier (1995), the following factors are associated with failure to control hypertension:

- Noncompliance on the part of patients with regard to medication and physician advice

- Physician satisfaction with suboptimal therapy

- Heterogeneous nature of the pathophysiology of hypertension, which makes it difficult to predict which patients will respond to a specific treatment

- Poor communication between physicians and patients

- Treatment guidelines that are too complex, theoretical, or otherwise unclear

Low patient compliance has been identified as one of the most important factors limiting the effectiveness of hypertension therapy (Lüscher, Vetter, Siegenthaler, and Vetter, 1985). As one might expect, treatment regimens requiring multiple daily doses and involving longer drug therapies can have a negative effect on patient compliance (Farmer, Jacobs, and Phillips, 1994). In addition, studies have shown that noncompliance occurs when the barriers of treatment (including side effects of medicines, disruption of lifestyle) to the patient are high (Richardson, Simons-Morton, and Annegers, 1993). Other factors that have a negative association with compliance include gender (males), age (youth), obesity, and cigarette smoking (Degoulet and others, 1983). Cultural beliefs about hypertension also may affect patient compliance with treatment regimens (Heurtin-Roberts and Reisin, 1992).

Health education interventions can increase compliance and can therefore affect the long-term control of hypertension (Levine, Green, and Morisky, 1987). Morisky and colleagues (1983) conducted a study to test three health education interventions for urban, poor, hypertensive patients: an exit interview immediately following a patient's encounter with a medical provider to reinforce the provider's instructions; a home visit to the patient to encourage family members to support the patient's treatment regimen; and invitations to small-group sessions designed to increase confidence and capacity to manage hypertension. Results after five years indicated that the three-part intervention had a positive effect on keeping appointments, controlling weight, and controlling blood pressure. In addition, compared with a control group that was not exposed to the health education series, patients in the intervention group demonstrated a slightly lower mortality rate.

Results from studies testing changes in diet as a mechanism to control hypertension have been mixed. For example, a nutritional-hygienic intervention program was able to reduce the incidence of hypertension, reduce sodium and alcohol intake, and increase physical activity (Stamler and others, 1989). In contrast, Davis and colleagues (1994) found that the use of a low-sodium, high-potassium diet was not effective as a practical therapeutic method to maintain blood pressure among an overweight population. Therefore, although it may not be effective as the sole treatment mechanism, dietary therapy may be an important adjunctive treatment in reducing cardiovascular risk (Oberman and others, 1990). The Treatment of Mild Hypertension Research Group (1991) found that nutritional-hygienic treatment, in conjunction with antihypertensive medication, reduced blood pressure to a much greater extent than nutritional-hygienic treatment alone.

Role of Primary Care and Specialist Physicians

Several studies have been conducted to determine whether outcomes for patients with hypertension vary by system of care or by generalist or subspecialist physician. One study by Greenfield and colleagues (1995) tested whether patient outcomes varied between health maintenance organizations, large multispecialty groups, or solo or single-specialty group practices. Using measurements of blood pressure and incidence of stroke after two years, four years, and seven years, the study did not yield any significant differences in health outcomes by care system or by physician specialty.

Similarly, a study by Adamson, Rodnick, and Guillion (1989) found no difference between family physicians and general internists with regard to treatment of hypertensive patients. The number and kinds of antihypertensive medications prescribed were similar, but internists performed more laboratory tests and were more likely to change medications than family physicians. In terms of patient outcome measures, however, Adamson and others found no difference in diastolic blood pressure, medication adherence, aerobic exercise, alcohol consumption, or dietary habits.

Treatment Teams

Dickinson and others (1981) developed an approach to identifying and treating hypertension patients based on a computer-generated feedback system to help identify poorly controlled patients, as well as a physician education program to enhance patient compliance. A follow-up evaluation found that feedback (reports to physicians containing information on clinical status of hypertensive patients) can increase the number of patient follow-up visits. The increased number of visits, however, did not appear to have a measurable effect on blood pressure control. None of these intervention mechanisms alone was found to have any impact on patient outcomes.

Schultz and Sheps (1994) have described a clinic-based model for managing outpatients with hypertension. Developed at the Mayo Clinic, this model uses a multidisciplinary team approach to care, which includes hypertension medical specialists, nurses, dietitians, and nurse-educators. The model was tested with three types of patients: short-term patients, those undergoing liver transplants, and long-term or continuing-care patients. An evaluation of the impact of this model found that all three treatment groups experienced success in a team-based program. Proponents of the model stress the importance of involving patients in managing their illness through cooperation, collaboration, and mutual respect among clinicians and patients.

Reduction in health care costs among hypertensive employees was observed through the use of a work-site monitoring and counseling program (Foote and Erfurt, 1991). A study evaluating the program found that the cost of health care claims were lower for employees in the intervention program than for those at the control site.

Conclusions

Hypertension, a major health problem in the United States, can be addressed through medication and lifestyle modification. Patient education relating to risk factor reduction, including dietary modifications, is essential to hypertension treatment. Team models for hypertension treatment appear promising, but relatively few model programs have been rigorously evaluated.

Stable Coronary Artery Disease

Coronary artery disease begins with a thickening of the coronary artery and eventually leads to plaque formation and localized narrowing in the coronary artery (Carbajal and Deedwania, 1995). In the past, it was generally assumed that patients suffering from stable angina constituted the largest group of patients with coronary artery disease. More recent studies report, however, that transient episodes of myocardial ischemia not associated with angina or other symptoms are the most common manifestation of coronary artery disease (Deedwania and Carbajal, 1990; Rocco and others, 1988; Stern and Tzivoni, 1974; Tzivoni and others, 1989).

According to one estimate, nearly 70 percent of the adult population is affected with some degree of coronary artery disease (Kingsley and Gupta, 1992), ranging from recurring angina attacks to sudden cardiac death (Carbajal and Deedwania, 1995). Deaths attributed to coronary artery disease have declined since the 1960s, apparently due to a reduction in coronary risk factors and improved medical care after acute myocardial infarction or onset of angina pectoris (Gillum, 1993; Gillum, Folsom, and Blackburn, 1984). Nevertheless, heart disease remains the leading cause of death in the United States (Gillum, 1993).

The morbidity and subsequent disability associated with coronary artery disease have far-reaching medical and socioeconomic implications. The approximately five hundred thousand coronary revascularization procedures performed each year in the United States, together with associated hospital stays, medications, medical personnel, and health care facility charges, result in costs of more than $50 billion (American Heart Association, 1993). The entire financial impact of cardiovascular disease in the United States is close to $135 billion (Centers for Disease Control and Prevention, 1992; Healthy People 2000, 1991).

The chief objectives for treating coronary artery disease include symptom relief with a minimum of side effects, enhancement of event-free survival, and risk factor control in order to reduce the disease's progression (Frye and others, 1989). When the condition is stable and not severe, treatment consists primarily of medical management and the reduction of modifiable risk factors. Medical treatment includes the use of three classes of drugs, either alone or in combination: beta-adrenergic blockers, calcium channel blockers, and nitrates. The decision about drug regimen, which also may include lipid-lowering drugs, is based on many factors, including patient characteristics, laboratory tests, and diagnostic strategies.

Patient Education

A meta-analysis of the impact of education on cardiac patients examined thirty-eight controlled studies of interventions to improve behavioral and clinical outcomes in patients with coronary heart disease (Mullen, Mains, and Velez, 1992). Although this was a study of cardiac patients, similar principles should apply to patients with stable coronary artery disease. The meta-analysis showed significant improvement in two important clinical outcomes: blood pressure and mortality. Morbidity and return-to-work were not significantly improved across studies, although patient education did seem to have a positive effect on return-to-work for some populations. Patient education was found to be effective for two behavioral outcomes—exercise and diet—but there was no significant effect found for smoking, medication adherence, or stress measures across studies. There were, however, positive effects for these behaviors when they were the primary targets of the intervention, as opposed to being incidental. Mullen and others concluded that cardiac patient education programs can have a measurable impact on blood pressure, mortality, exercise, and diet, and that other outcomes may also be affected positively. They recommended that cardiac education programs use reinforcement, give feedback, offer opportunity for individualization, facilitate behavior change through skills and resources, and recognize varying patient needs and abilities.

Treatment Teams

Because one major treatment goal—reduction of modifiable risk factors—requires active participation and cooperation on the part of the patient and family in a number of areas (diet, exercise, treatment adherence, and stress reduction), a team approach to managing stable coronary artery disease would appear desirable. Such an approach would coordinate treatment provided by the primary care physician and cardiologist; the services of nurses, dietitians, and exercise therapists; and the efforts of patients and family members. There does not appear to be any literature, however, that specifically evaluates team management of stable coronary artery disease. Nonetheless, components of a possible team approach to management are described in the literature.

A nurse, practicing in a variety of settings, can play a major role in helping people assume responsibility for their health behaviors; the goal would be to prevent the development and progression of coronary artery disease (Stovsky, 1992). Secondary prevention applies to patients who already have stable coronary artery disease. Although secondary prevention strategies may begin in the hospital, recall of information received in the hospital is often poor. Hence, it is especially important to reinforce information through patient follow-up in the outpatient area. There, the nurse can provide emotional support, assess exercise tolerance and patient motivation, and help to modify goals and interventions as needed. The nurse also can communicate healthy behaviors and document changes in patient functional status and progress toward goal achievement. As the nurse conveys this information to other members of the health care team, including the patient, it will reinforce positive behavior (Parchert and Simon, 1988).

The cardiologist is certain to be a member of the health care team for patients with stable coronary artery disease. A dietitian also may have a place on the team to advise the patient on altering eating patterns in order to lower lipids and achieve weight goals.

Smoking cessation specialists may be helpful, and the neighborhood health club can play an important role in facilitating an exercise regimen for patients with stable coronary artery disease.

The health care team typically encompasses a variety of individuals, but the major responsibility for the care of patients with stable coronary artery disease rests with the primary care physician and the cardiologist. Guidelines for the treatment of stable coronary artery disease are a tool for the primary care physician, both for ongoing management of the disease and for referral to other health care professionals. Using guidelines may enable the primary care physician to handle most of the stable patient's routine care and to avoid many costly referrals to the cardiologist (Institute for Clinical Systems Integration, 1995). To date, there has not been an evaluation of the effectiveness of specific practice guidelines in this area.

Social support often plays an important role in the treatment of stable coronary artery disease. A recent study evaluated how three types of social support (informational, emotional, and tangible) from the spouse and health care provider affected both short-term and long-term recovery outcomes for males following cardiac illness (Yates, 1995). Greater satisfaction with health care provider support was associated with improvement in short- and long-term physical recovery. Tangible aid, that is, help with the activities of daily living, from the spouse was associated with better short-term psychological recovery. Satisfaction with the spouse's emotional support was associated with better short- and long-term psychological recovery outcomes. Lack of social support from the spouse was associated with depressive symptoms. These findings highlight the importance of different sources and types of social support on both physical and psychological recovery outcomes in male cardiac patients.

Conclusions

Stable coronary artery disease affects a large proportion of the population and has immense consequences in terms of morbidity, mortality, and direct and indirect costs to society. Because treatment is complex and multifaceted, and because its effectiveness is influenced by patient behaviors and social support, a team approach to care would appear appropriate. There seems to be no published research that evaluates such an approach, however.

Implications for Improving Chronic Illness Management

The difficulties in implementing and evaluating innovative "model" treatment programs, and in ultimately drawing conclusions from them, are well known. In summarizing these difficulties, Keith (1991, p. 272) observes that "trying out new treatment models entails some risk. First, such models are apt to collide with current conceptions about acceptable professional practice. Second, if they address the problem of costs, they may result in staff reductions and decreases in revenue. Third, to establish the utility of alternative methods, a research commitment of considerable proportion is necessary." Keith concludes that "demonstrating the effectiveness of team functioning is complicated, because the problem is both clinical *and organizational*" (emphasis added, p. 271).

With some notable exceptions, the research studies described in this section have focused on clinical issues. They have several points in common:

- The patient's central role in the management of chronic illnesses is acknowledged in most models and studies. There is substantial emphasis placed on patient education and patient self-management, with the exact nature of these activities varying across different models and illnesses.

- It is common for chronic illness management models to use a team approach to care. The team model usually emphasizes the role of a nurse-coordinator, who interacts on a regular basis with patients as a clinician, an educator, and a link to medical and social services. In general, the resources involved in implementing the different variations of this model have not been carefully documented.

• Although most chronic illness evolves over a substantial period of time and can be characterized by gradual deterioration in functioning with acute flare-ups of symptoms, most research studies have measured outcomes over relatively short time spans.

When organizational issues are identified in the clinical research literature, they are often introduced as post hoc explanations for why specific models may not have demonstrated the anticipated degree of clinical effectiveness. This suggests that a better understanding of the organizational and managerial dimensions of chronic illness treatment could help identify determinants of model performance.

4

Learning from Management Models

In Chapter Three, we reviewed the literature on models for chronic illness treatment and concluded that in their design and implementation, relatively little attention had been paid to organizational and managerial issues. Apparently, these issues were not considered sufficiently germane to model performance to be addressed in the model description or incorporated in the research design. In this chapter, we attempt to provide insight into the potential influence of organizational issues by drawing on the general literature about organizations.

The health care team has an analogue in this literature—the work group. We will develop the general concept of the work group and examine its internal and external relationships, applying these concepts to chronic illness management teams. Then we will summarize two articles on work groups in acute care settings and discuss the articles' implications for improving chronic illness management.

The Work Group Concept

In organizational literature, organizations have been described as "cooperative systems," "institutions," "decision-making systems," and, less formally, as "systems for getting work done" (Perrow, 1967). Most health care professionals participate in formal health care delivery systems or organizations that often define the management of chronic illnesses as one of their activities. As earlier chapters have noted, an important characteristic of chronic illnesses is that patients and their families usually play significant roles in managing the illness, even though they are not formally linked to the organization through employment or other contractual means. Circumstances of this nature have long been recognized in the organizational literature. Parsons (1961) noted that professional services can exhibit a "very important pattern where the recipient of the service becomes an operative member of the service-providing organization" (p. 39). Furthermore, according to Parsons (1961) and Thompson (1967), the recipient's role can have important implications for the design and functioning of these organizations.

Organizations that involve clients in the production of services have been called *therapeutic* or *inductive organizations*, because they effectively "induct" the client into the organization. Thus, health care delivery systems that participate in the management of chronic illnesses can be characterized as *inductive organizations*, in which the patient and family are "operative members" of the organization.

A central problem organizations face is how to organize the available resources in order to carry out the organization's work. Usually, there is a great deal of uncertainty about the nature of the work that needs to be done and how best to accomplish that work. Not infrequently, there is even uncertainty about how to determine if the work has been accomplished successfully (Thompson, 1967). The different means by which organizations accomplish work have been the subject of extensive analysis. An approach that appears particularly relevant for the management of chronic illnesses, and one that is closely related to the concept of the health care team, is that of the work group. Indeed, organizational literature often refers to health care teams to illustrate the design and function of work groups.

Hetherington and Rundall (1983) observe that "it is difficult to think of a substantial task within our modern health service organizations that does not require a team, or work group, for its completion" (p. 167). Hetherington and Rundall describe a *work group* as consisting of "two or more individuals who voluntarily interact in a task-oriented situation in such a manner that the behavior and/or performance of each group member is influenced to some extent by the behavior and/or performance of other members" (p. 171).

This is similar to Halstead's (1976) definition of a *health care team* as "a group of two or more health professionals from different disciplines who share common values and work toward common objectives" (p. 508). In the treatment of a chronic illness, the work group can be viewed as including health professionals (who are formal members of the traditional health care team) and the patient and family (who are "inducted" into the organization).

Several interrelated factors that are internal to the chronic illness work group are likely to influence its functioning in complex ways. These factors, as identified in the literature on work groups, include the group's social structure, the processes used to carry out the work (for example, provide the treatment), and the ways in which the group chooses to assess its effectiveness (Hetherington and Rundall, 1983, p. 173).

The work group does not function in isolation, though. These factors and their interrelationships are affected by the work group's environment. To simplify our discussion, let us assume that the work group can do little, if anything, to modify its external environment. As identified in the literature, external characteristics that affect how work groups function include the following:

- The nature of the work to be done (which presumably is heavily influenced by the nature of the chronic disease to be treated)

- The characteristics of the organization in which the work group is embedded (for example, its culture, the scale of its operations, and the quality of its support systems)

- The characteristics of the larger environment (for example, payer expectations, regulations, practice norms, and reimbursement mechanisms)

The complex relationships of characteristics within a work group and between the work group and its external environment are depicted in Figure 4.1. This chapter will now discuss the different components of Figure 4.1 in greater detail, beginning with the dynamics in a work group and then examining its external environment.

Relationships Within Work Groups

A work group's structure is typically discussed using concepts such as status, roles, norms, and size (Hetherington and Rundall, 1983). *Status* is defined as a person's position within a social system. For instance, specialists would presumably enjoy a certain status in a chronic illness work group because they have specialized knowledge. Associated with that status is an expected set of behaviors, constituting the specialist's *role* on the team. *Norms* are the generalized behavioral expectations that apply to team members. For instance, as a result of her status and role, a specialist might be expected to make a definitive diagnosis about a patient's chronic illness. The work group's *size* is defined as the number of individuals involved in carrying out the work.

The processes used to perform work within groups are described in the literature using concepts such as leadership, communication, and coordination (for example, see Bettenhausen, 1991). The term *leadership* can encompass a broad set of behaviors. At one level, it involves setting goals and planning for the work group, as well as promoting and protecting group values (Burns and Becker, 1983, p. 146). At another level, *leadership* refers to the more mundane issues relating to organizing work flows, solving production problems, and motivating other work group members to perform tasks.

Figure 4.1. The Work Group and Its Environment.

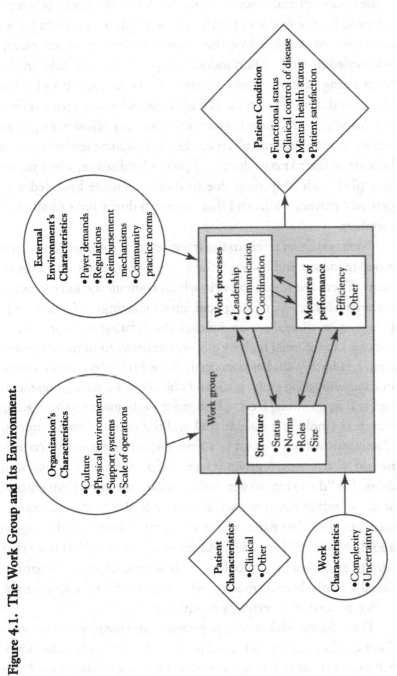

Source: Institute for Research and Education.

Some organizational theorists argue that *leadership* should be a term reserved for the first set of activities, whereas *management* better describes the second. In either case, the concept of leadership acknowledges that certain individuals play dominant roles in the functioning of work groups. It raises questions about how leaders obtain and sustain positions of leadership, what constitutes effective leadership, and how leaders' activities vary across work groups and over time. For example, specialists may assume leadership roles because of their knowledge about particular diseases, while nurses may play leadership roles due to their extensive knowledge of patients' current status and their (nurses') direct links to all team members.

Communication refers to the transmittal of information among group members and between the group and its external environment. There are various ways in which communication can occur within a work group, ranging from formal meetings and memoranda (focusing on clinical or nonclinical issues relating to chronically ill patients) to informal hallway discussions between nurse and physician. Leadership studies commonly focus on leaders' effectiveness in communicating group goals and objectives to work group members and in providing feedback on group performance to both group members (including the patient) and the external environment. Communication is viewed as a key to achieving effective coordination within a work group (Hage, 1983). *Coordination* has been defined as "the extent to which the various interdependent parts of an organization function each according to the needs and requirements of the other parts, and of the total system" (Hetherington and Rundall, 1983, p. 189). March and Simon (1958) note that coordination is a basic problem in all organizations and organizational subunits because much of what the organization does cannot be determined with certainty in advance.

They distinguish between *programmed* and *nonprogrammed* coordination. In programmed coordination, control over production is achieved primarily through planning or through having predetermined protocols. An example would be treatment protocols that specify which chronic illness work group members are to take which actions under different circumstances. Because one cannot predict how some patients with chronic illnesses will respond to treatment, however, other means of coordination are likely to be required, as well.

When the unexpected occurs, work group members need non-programmed coordination so that they can adjust to the new situation. For instance, a patient might communicate to other members a change in his condition that would lead to change in the team's activities. In most discussions of work groups, the degree and quality of the coordination are seen as important predictors of the work group's ability to achieve its objectives.

A third recognized component of work groups is the set of measures used to assess performance (Shortell and Kalvzny, 1983). Most work groups assess performance by measuring efficiency, although the exact definition of that measure can vary. For instance, the work group may define *efficiency* as the degree to which a specified treatment goal is attained with a given allocation of resources. Alternatively, it may define *efficiency* as the degree to which routine tasks are completed using as few resources as possible. A number of other efficiency measures are possible, with the choice of measures likely to be influenced by the group's structure and work processes.

Many authors have also noted the prevalence of performance measures that are not related to efficiency, such as the degree to which the group achieves a common culture or a high level of morale. (See Wall and Nolan, 1986, 1987, or Wall, Galanes, and Love, 1987, for an analysis of member satisfaction and conflict in work groups.) Groups sometimes view these measures as being intrinsically important; other groups see them as being valuable because they can enhance efficiency.

Most likely, all of these internal components of work groups are not only related but also simultaneously determined. That is, while the group's structure influences its work processes and the way it measures its performance, reciprocal relationships are also likely. The group's assessment of performance affects the way it performs its activities and the group's structure. (For example, such measures influence the status of different group members and their roles within the group.) Similarly, the way the group coordinates its activities can influence its structure and the performance measures it adopts.

The Importance of the External Environment

The relationships within a work group are themselves shaped by the group's external environment. In particular, three features of the external environment can affect a group: those related to the work to be performed, those related to the organization in which the work group is located, and those reflecting the larger world in which the work group and organization function.

Characteristics of the Group's Work

Terms commonly used to describe work may also help to discern the types of work required for different chronic diseases. For instance, in the terminology of Hetherington and Rundall (1983), *complexity* refers to the number of different items or tasks that a work group must accomplish simultaneously. The larger the number of required tasks, the more complex the work is. Others have used *complexity* to refer to the amount of knowledge needed to carry out the work or the difficulty of the tasks performed.

Closely related to the notion of *complexity* is that of *uncertainty*. In its most common use, *uncertainty* refers to the degree to which there is not a known, predictable relationship between activities (for example, treatment provided for the patient) and outcomes (for example, the degree to which clinical indicators of the patient's health status improve). The less predictable the relationship, the more uncertain the work is.

The complexity and uncertainty of the work performed in managing a chronic illness will likely influence the work group's structure, work process, and even its measures of performance (David, Randolph, and Pearce, 1989). Most of the time, this work would appear to involve both considerable complexity and uncertainty, but these aspects may vary, depending on the nature and progression of the disease and clinical approaches to treatment.

Characteristics of the Organizational Environment

The clinicians and social service professionals in a work group treating chronic illnesses often belong to different organizations. The way in which a work group functions is likely to reflect the influences of these "parent" organizations on work group members. If various parent organizations have different cultures or revenue needs, this could lead to conflicting goals for the work group and conflicts among work group members over roles and norms.

Even when all the group members belong to the same organization, that organization's characteristics will likely affect the group's functioning. For instance, chronic illness group members in a large managed care organization might adopt an explicit "population-based" approach to chronic illness management, with an emphasis on achieving the greatest good for the greatest number of enrollees within a fixed budget. In contrast, if a chronic illness management work group is based in a clinic and relies on fee-for-service revenues to finance its operations, it might try giving maximum care to each patient; it will be constrained, however, by the boundaries of acceptable practice and rules about which services insurers will cover. In a third scenario, a work group located within an organization that is actively trying to develop and use clinical guidelines might try to incorporate guidelines in the treatment of chronic illness; this group would be more likely to do so (in part, to fit with the prevailing organizational culture) than would a chronic illness work group in an organization that makes minimal use of guidelines.

Characteristics of the Larger Environment

Both the chronic illness work group and its parent organization function within a larger environment. The characteristics of this larger environment—whether defined at the community, state, or national level—can influence the way a work group organizes and carries out its activities (Walsh and McPhee, 1992). For instance, practice norms regarding the treatment of a chronic illness can vary across communities in ways that influence the roles of specialists, primary care physicians, and nurses within work groups. Similarly, variations in the availability of social services across communities could influence the degree to which treatment plans incorporate such providers. At the state level, variation in mandated insurance coverage could influence the sorts of services delivered as part of the chronic illness treatment, and variation in licensure requirements could influence the types of clinical personnel involved in the treatment.

Acute Care Models of Work Groups

There have been some recent attempts to describe and assess work groups in acute care settings. Two articles in this area are particularly notable because of their implications for chronic illness management. The first addresses team care in an emergency room, and the second describes how "temporary firms" emerge in community hospital settings.

Emergency Rooms

Argote (1982) offers a theoretical and empirical analysis of how personnel in hospital emergency rooms operate under various levels of "input uncertainty." By *input uncertainty*, she means the number of possibilities in a given situation and the probability that these various scenarios will occur. In her study, "patients in various conditions" (p. 422) constitute these possibilities. Uncertainty is considered to be greatest when there are many alternatives and when they are equally likely to occur.

Argote then draws on previous studies to develop hypotheses about the relationships between (1) uncertainty and measures of organizational coordination and (2) means of coordination and measures of organizational effectiveness. She points out that coordination can be achieved through a variety of means, but there are two basic types of coordination: programmed and nonprogrammed. Programmed coordination occurs when "the activities of organization members are dictated by plans, programs, and relationships specified in advance by the organization. . . . In nonprogrammed coordination, activities are not specified in advance by the organization, but rather are worked out on the spot by organization members" (p. 423).

Argote hypothesizes that emergency rooms will rely on programmed means of coordination when uncertainty is low and on nonprogrammed means when uncertainty is high. Thus, she believes that as uncertainty varies in emergency rooms, approaches to coordination also vary. She also hypothesizes that programmed coordination methods will increase organizational effectiveness more when input uncertainty is low; accordingly, nonprogrammed coordination will enhance effectiveness more when uncertainty is high. One of her measures of effectiveness is how quickly an emergency unit responds to a particular admission.

In Argote's analysis of emergency rooms' coordination of work, two features have limited relevance for chronic disease management. First, she adopts a standard input-transformation-output work cycle in discussing the emergency unit's operations. The patient who is "input" is "transformed" through the emergency treatment received and is then discharged as "output." This may be a useful way to structure discussion in an acute care setting, in which a cure is the goal of treatment. It does not, however, adequately characterize the process of chronic illness management, because in that situation a patient is not expected to be "discharged." In contrast, the "transformation" or "throughput" phase of the work cycle is expected to be ongoing. Therefore, the treatment team's activities must be organized to optimize patient outcomes over time, not to respond to a single event.

Argote's discussion of programmed and nonprogrammed methods of coordination would seem to have more relevance to the management of chronic illnesses. To the degree that there is considerable uncertainty with respect to the patient's condition at any time (many alternatives are equally likely to occur), the treatment team would be expected to adopt relatively nonprogrammed means of coordination. Individual treatment team members would need to respond on the spot to changed conditions. For example, a patient might have considerable power to adjust medication dosages as she experiences more or less pain. In contrast, when changes in patient condition are more easily categorized and characterized, it may be possible to achieve effective coordination in the work group through the use of more programmed approaches. For instance, a man with asthma might adjust his medication when self-administered peak-flow meter readings reached predetermined levels, and he might enlist other team members' help if prespecified responses to medication adjustments did not occur.

Temporary Firms in Community Hospitals

In a second article of interest, Chilingerian and Glavin (1994) have developed a model of clinical services provided in a community hospital. In this model, the physician is portrayed as the manager of a "temporary-firm" (T-firm) that "emerges and operates every time that physician admits and cares for a patient in the hospital. This model builds on the idea of the attending physician as the principal decision-maker and gatekeeper to the production of a hospital's clinical services. However, it also brings the relationships between the attending physician and other hospital caregivers into a new light" (p. 291).

An important feature of the T-firm model is its emphasis on the temporary nature of treatment teams that form to provide acute care for patients. This impermanence causes particular problems in the management of care: "Temporary relationships mean that communication, coordination and control are more difficult, and subsequent outcomes may be less efficient" (p. 291).

In addition, the T-firm model explicitly views the physician as the chief decision maker. In the acute care setting, according to Chilingerian and Glavin, "Caregivers vary in the amount of time and attention they provide to a given patient, and the individual caregivers may change from day to day. Thus, there are only two stable elements in the T-firm—the hospitalized patient(s) and the attending physician" (p. 296).

This scenario is complicated, in their minds, by the "trained incapacity" (p. 300) of physicians to think and act like managers. Recognizing this, hospital administrators attempt to provide substitutes for leadership in the form of standardized treatment protocols and semipermanent work teams. Chilingerian and Glavin use the T-firm to develop hypotheses about the factors that could affect T-firm efficiency, but they do not test these hypotheses empirically.

The Chilingerian and Glavin analysis underscores again an important difference between the treatment of acute and chronic illness—the first is short term, and the second is not. This is particularly evident in the authors' description of acute care treatment teams as extremely unstable. In contrast, chronic care treatment teams have the potential to be relatively stable over time. For them, miscommunication may be less of a problem than in the T-firms described by Chilingerian and Glavin.

Implications for Improving Chronic Illness Management

The work group concept is commonly used to describe how work is accomplished within organizations. It is also a familiar concept in health care literature, where it frequently surfaces in discussions of health care teams. Work groups can have complex structures and communication requirements. Effectively coordinating the activities of work group members can be difficult, particularly when goals conflict or are not clearly defined. Furthermore, work groups' performance is likely to be influenced by a variety of factors outside their immediate control. These include the nature of the work to be performed, the characteristics of the organizations in which group members function, and features of the environment outside work groups. The concept of a work group, as developed in the organizational and management literature, provides an attractive framework for discussing how, in theory, the "work" of caring for chronic illness ought to be organized and performed.

The two articles that apply the work group concept to acute care highlight differences between acute and chronic illnesses—differences that affect the way treatment is organized. The first obvious difference relates to the work group's stability, which in turn relates to the nature of acute versus chronic illness. Many of the challenges in delivering acute care, as described in these articles, concern the very temporary status of work groups. For example, because groups form for brief periods and then disband, there is little opportunity to explore variations in group members' roles. In contrast, when the illness is long term, there is at least the opportunity to adjust group members' roles as the illness changes. Plus, there is a chance to educate the patient and the family about the illness and to define roles for them as part of the work group.

A second difference relates to the work group's leadership. In the acute care settings discussed in these two articles, there is no ambiguity about leadership—a physician plays the dominant role in treating the illness, and the rest of the work group is assembled primarily to support the physician. Again, the nature of chronic versus acute illness suggests that the role of the physician—whether specialist or generalist—is likely to be considerably more fluid in the treatment of chronic illness. As a chronic illness progresses, the patient or clinician-coordinator may sometimes play a dominant role in coordinating and managing treatment, whereas at other times (for instance, during acute flare-ups) the physician will be clearly in charge.

5

Challenges in Applying
Work Group Models

In Chapter Four, we introduced the concept of the work group, discussed how work groups function in the abstract, and summarized two studies of work groups in acute care settings. In this chapter, we will relate that discussion to the treatment of chronic illnesses. We will organize this discussion by the issues identified in Chapters Two and Three: the longitudinal nature of chronic illnesses in which cures in the acute care sense are generally not possible, the central role of patients and families in managing chronic illnesses, the large number of individuals and variety of resources typically involved in the management of chronic illnesses, and the difficulty of determining whether treatment processes have been successful. Finally, we will discuss the implications of these issues for chronic illness work group design and operations.

The Longitudinal Nature of Chronic Illness:
Impact on Group Development

By definition, "chronic" illnesses last for substantial periods of time. This means that work group development or maturation over time has bearing on how groups approach the treatment of chronic illness.

The literature on the treatment of chronic illness suggests that a predictable sequence of activities usually occurs. As described previously, this sequence involves diagnosis, development of a treatment plan, implementation of the treatment plan, and evaluation of the treatment's impact on the patient, with possible reevaluation of the diagnosis or reconfiguration of the treatment plan.

This linear conceptualization of the treatment of chronic illness has a clear counterpart in the organizational literature on the development of groups in general, and work groups in particular (for example, Gersick, 1988; Pearce and Ravlin, 1987). For instance, Hare (1976) describes work group development as consisting of the following stages: defining the situation, developing new skills, developing appropriate roles, and carrying out the work. Lacoursiere (1980) assigns the following labels to the stages of work group development: orientation, dissatisfaction, resolution, production, and termination. In more descriptive language, McGrath (1984) observes that groups (1) generate plans, ideas, and goals, (2) choose or agree on alternatives, goals, and policies, (3) resolve conflicts and develop norms, and (4) perform tasks and maintain cohesion.

Not only is work group development similar to chronic illness management in its linear structure, as conceptualized by these authors, but its stages are also generally consistent with the activities of chronic illness management. The group development dynamic proposed by Lacoursiere (1980) illustrates this point.

In the orientation stage, group members have positive expectations about the group but are concerned about how it will function and what their roles will be. The group attempts to define goals and tasks and allocate work to group members. With respect to chronic illness management, this corresponds to the diagnosis of the disease and the development of the care plan. During this stage, group members (including the patient) define their roles and receive task assignments. As the team reaches a diagnosis and creates a plan, the patient develops positive expectations, feeling more confident that things will improve.

As described by Lacoursiere (1980), a critical dissatisfaction stage often follows the initial orientation stage in group development. Dissatisfaction occurs when the reality of the group experience does not meet group members' expectations. This dissonance may emerge because tasks are more difficult to accomplish or take longer than expected, causing group members to feel incompetent or confused. In that case, group members may have to develop certain skills before performing assigned tasks, and this process may be slower than expected. Frustrated group members may repudiate the leader's authority or challenge the roles of other group members. Some groups can become stuck in this stage and never succeed in accomplishing their work effectively. To the degree that most or all work groups experience a dissatisfaction stage, there are potentially important implications for chronic disease work groups.

In the treatment of a chronic disease, the dissatisfaction stage seems most likely to occur shortly after the group initiates the treatment plan. The plan may ask the patient to play a much more important and intensive role in managing the illness than he or she expected. This could include taking blood samples, giving injections, manipulating peak-flow meters, and changing exercise and dietary habits. Some of these self-care activities may require skills that patients do not possess. In addition, there will likely be much less interaction with medical care providers than during the orientation stage, and there may be no immediate, noticeable improvement in patient functioning or symptoms. As a result, patients may feel abandoned by the medical care system, uncertain about whether they are doing "the right thing," and resentful of the demands that the treatment plan has imposed on them, particularly when it requires major lifestyle changes.

Once this particular dynamic of work group development has been acknowledged, the challenge is to minimize the time that the work group spends in the dissatisfaction stage, as well as the possibility that it will become stuck in this stage. The dissatisfaction stage arises when expectations exceed what can realistically be accomplished. For this reason, it is important for the work group to develop implementation plans that both the patient and the clinicians find realistic. These plans must be communicated clearly to all group members. Work group members (in most cases, patients) who will be called on to practice new skills must receive adequate training. For the plan to be realistic, the goals and task assignments must be tailored to individual patients, who will enter the chronic illness management process with different physical and mental capabilities and varying social support systems. Work group members (particularly patients and clinicians) must maintain regular contact so as to detect and address feelings of frustration and resentment in their early stages of development.

Work groups that do progress beyond dissatisfaction move into the resolution stage. The tension between initial high expectations and the reality of what can reasonably be accomplished dissipates, primarily because group members recalibrate their expectations. Clinicians become more realistic about patients' skill levels and commitment to the treatment plan, given their compliance with making changes in their lives. Patients become more realistic about the treatment's potential to alleviate symptoms and improve functioning. As their skill levels increase, they become more confident, and their self-care activities become more productive. Group members become more comfortable in their relationships with each other and with their roles in the group.

In the production stage, the group functions at its most efficient level. Group members carry out their tasks with relative autonomy. When needed, however, they are able to communicate easily with each other. In a chronic illness management work group, patients readily contact clinicians with questions about treatment, medication side effects, or unexpected changes in symptoms. Providers become more knowledgeable about the patient's broader life and are able to suggest social support services to enhance treatment effectiveness. All members understand and accept group roles and norms. The group's high levels of production enhance feelings of competence and satisfaction.

Sustaining these feelings is a critical part of maintaining the production stage. Toward this end, the group can take specific steps, including scheduling regular opportunities for communication; giving group members continuing educational opportunities about disease processes, medications, skill development, and the like; and reaffirming group roles and norms through feedback about performance.

Although groups are usually portrayed as evolving in this linear manner, in part for ease of exposition, more recent literature (for example, Gersick, 1988; Bettenhausen, 1991) recognizes that the different stages of group development can overlap and that the transition from one stage to another may not be distinct. Furthermore, intervening events can cause the group to regress to a previous stage of development or, in the extreme, to dissolve. For example, introducing a new member into a work group can result in a redefinition of norms and roles, moving the group to the dissatisfaction or even the orientation stage. An externally imposed change in work group objectives or organizational support can have similar effects.

In the context of a chronic illness management work group, the group's composition is most likely to change when a clinician withdraws from the group. This can happen if clinicians change employment or if organizations change strategies for treating chronic illnesses. In this scenario, roles and relationships will need to be renegotiated, but the group may be able to return quickly to the production stage. If the group changes because the patient withdraws or changes insurance coverage in a way that limits work group activities, the entire group development process is likely to begin anew in a different medical care organization but may be facilitated by the skills that the patient has developed through participation in previous chronic illness management work groups.

Some degree of discontinuity in group development is inevitable. The most common externally imposed change affecting chronic illness management work groups is an abrupt alteration in the patient's health status. Although the long-term course of most chronic illnesses is relatively predictable, there can be dramatic short-term fluctuations in disease symptoms. It is also relatively common for patients with chronic diseases to develop comorbid conditions that must be treated in conjunction with the chronic illness.

Under these circumstances, the chronic illness management work group is likely to move back to the orientation stage. The group composition will need to be reexamined, as will members' roles. New skills may need to be developed or introduced into the group through the incorporation of new members. If group members do not recognize that they need to move back to an orientation stage, the group may wallow in a dissatisfaction stage in which treatment is no longer perceived as effective. Group members may blame each other for failing to perform assigned roles or may become confused and frustrated. This can be avoided if group members are able to detect changes in a patient's condition and accurately assess their importance for the work group. Such a productive intervention is most likely to occur if members have established good communication.

Patients' Central Role in Managing Chronic Illness

When a patient becomes a work group member, the group must create explicit roles and norms about the patient's participation. Such clearly defined roles enable the patient to work with other group members to achieve a consensual set of objectives. These roles and norms must be communicated effectively within the work group and adjusted for any changes in the patient's needs and desires, as well as changes in the group's composition or external environment.

How can a group achieve these tasks effectively? That is, how can a group integrate the patient as a member and ensure effective patient participation in the group's work as conditions change over time? Very little of the literature on work groups addresses this issue. There are, however, numerous published articles on work groups' dynamics, especially about the way in which groups accomplish work within organizations and the problem of motivating work group members. This branch of the work group literature mainly discusses the problems of managing work groups when members work for a single organization (but frequently come from different organizational subunits). Nevertheless, the literature does identify concepts that appear highly relevant for chronic illness management teams in which patients play prominent roles.

Rather than attempting to summarize this extensive literature, the discussion that follows focuses on one article that integrates the concept of situational leadership with the development and functioning of work groups (Carew, Parisi-Carew, and Blanchard, 1986). The justification for this singular focus is that the authors' recommendations have relatively clear and direct implications for the incorporation and continued involvement of chronically ill patients in their own care.

The concept of situational leadership assumes that there are different leadership styles and that these styles are likely to vary in their effectiveness, depending on the circumstances. Two broad dimensions of leadership behavior are identified as "directive" and "supportive." Leadership is highly directive if, among other things, it emphasizes one-way communication with others and close supervision of work activities. It is highly supportive if the leader provides support and encouragement and involves others in decision making.

These two concepts can be used to describe four different leadership styles. A "directing" leader exhibits highly directive behavior with little emphasis on supportive behavior. Directing leaders articulate goals, provide clear instructions for achieving those goals, and closely supervise work activity. "Coaching" leaders are both highly directive and highly supportive; they articulate goals and tasks but also are open to others' suggestions and ideas. "Supporting" leaders are highly supportive with few directive behaviors. They incorporate others in setting goals and defining tasks and actively offer their support in carrying out these tasks. Finally, "delegating" leaders are neither highly supportive nor highly directive. They turn over responsibility to others, who are assumed to be able to provide their own motivation and direction.

Which leadership style to employ in any situation is supposed to depend heavily on group members' levels of competence and commitment. To simplify their arguments, Carew, Parisi-Carew, and Blanchard (1986) identify four developmental levels:

- High competence, high commitment

- High competence, variable commitment

- Some competence, low commitment

- Low competence, high commitment

They believe that each leadership style is most appropriate for one of these developmental stages. When group members show high competence and commitment, a delegating style of leadership is likely to be effective. When competence is high but commitment is not, a supporting leadership style is necessary. If commitment is questionable and competence is low, a coaching style is more appropriate, as workers require direction, close supervision, and encouragement. When competence is low but commitment is high, a directing style is likely to achieve the best results.

Carew, Parisi-Carew, and Blanchard's work (1986) can help chronic illness work groups develop effective approaches for involving patients in their own care. In addition, these authors make a major contribution by marrying their ideas about situational leadership with the aforementioned stages of work group development.

They argue that a directing style of leadership is needed in the orientation stage. At this stage in a chronic illness work group, group members are likely to be quite committed, particularly patients. Conversely, patients' skill levels are likely to be low. Patients need to have group roles and goals clearly articulated, they need to be instructed in how to perform their tasks, and they need to be closely supervised to ensure that they have achieved the appropriate level of technical skill.

According to Carew, Parisi-Carew, and Blanchard, a "coaching" style of leadership is likely to be more effective than other styles in the dissatisfaction stage of group development. Although the patient has achieved some degree of competence, morale and commitment have declined as initial expectations have failed to be met. Not only should attention continue to be paid to building skills but patients' dissatisfaction with initial results must also be acknowledged and addressed. This requires an approach that combines direction with support.

If the work group moves to the resolution stage, supporting leadership is required to facilitate patient participation in the work group. The emphasis should be on developing a partnership with the patient and on acknowledging patient accomplishments in managing the treatment of the illness.

Finally, in the production stage, it may be possible to adopt a delegating style of leadership. The patient's competence and commitment are high, and a clinician-leader must show that she trusts the patient to perform tasks effectively. The clinician may find this style of leadership difficult, as it may diminish her perceived "special status" in the work group.

It is important for the leader to acknowledge that different styles of interacting with patients in groups will likely yield different results, depending on the group's stage of development. This understanding will help the leader develop and sustain effective patient involvement over time. Translating this observation into action is not straightforward, however. It requires that work group leaders be trained in group dynamics and in alternative leadership approaches. It also requires that leaders be able to alter their approaches in response to different stages of group development and different levels of patient skills.

Coordinating Group Efforts

As described above, many different individuals may be involved in the management of any chronic illness, including the patient, the patient's family, a primary care physician, a specialist, a nurse, and at least one social service provider. Each of these individuals is expected to contribute specific resources or expertise to the work group. As Charns (1983, p. 211) notes, "When interconnected elements of work are performed by different people, components must be coordinated to ensure effective performance. Coordination requires resources from the organization, such as development and use of plans and protocols, supervision of people responsible for interconnected elements, or discussion among these people."

In most work groups, it is assumed that effective coordination can be achieved primarily through informal mechanisms and with little conscious effort, because a small number of members work in close proximity and therefore have continuous interaction. This is not likely to be a safe assumption with respect to chronic illness management work groups. The group members carry out many of their individual tasks when other members are not present. Sometimes they do so in physically separate locations. For example, the diabetes patient may complete blood glucose readings at home, the physician may assess the patient's condition at the office without other work group members present, and the nurse may monitor the patient's condition through telephone conversations that do not involve other work group members. In this situation, it may not be reasonable to expect that work group activities will be coordinated through ongoing, informal interactions in the work setting. This problem is compounded by the relatively large number of participants in a chronic illness management work group. As the work group size increases, so do the possible channels for communication and interaction. As Charns and Schaefer (1983) note, a doubling of group size from three to six members results in a fivefold increase in possible interactions.

These characteristics of chronic illness management work groups suggest that a conscious strategy is needed to achieve effective coordination within the work group, and that resources will need to be allocated to implement this strategy. The general literature on organizations has identified a variety of approaches to coordinating work. As we mentioned in Chapter Four, March and Simon (1958) suggested two broad types of coordination—programmed and nonprogrammed. Programmed coordination involves coordinating work activities through a formal, usually written plan. Nonprogrammed coordination is essentially coordination by feedback, with work group members communicating with each other when events deviate from expectations.

Some researchers have characterized programmed coordination (especially if written) as "formal" and nonprogrammed coordination as "informal." Formal, programmed methods of coordination are expected to be more effective when work groups are large and when members' tasks have a low level of complexity and uncertainty. That is, formal methods work if the tasks are relatively routine and if there is a predictable relationship between performing each task and an outcome. There is much in chronic disease management that fits this description. For instance, for asthma patients to take and record peak-flow readings is a relatively routine task, as is the nurse's periodic telephone assessments of the patient's condition or the social service provider's provision of help with bathing or transportation.

There are just as clearly tasks in chronic illness management that do not fit this mold, however. For instance, the diagnosis of diseases of the joint and the prescription of the appropriate medication is not an easily "programmable" task but rather one that exhibits a high degree of complexity and uncertainty. Similarly, the clinician's response to an acute exacerbation of chronic disease symptoms may require substantial informal coordination.

This suggests that the chronic illness management work group will need to adopt both programmed and nonprogrammed means of coordination, making conscious decisions about when each type of coordinating activity is likely to be most effective. This may require the group to establish what Hetherington and Rundall (1983) have termed *liaison roles*. These are "special roles created to help coordinate the work of group members and to resolve conflicts among them" (p. 179).

Charns and Schaefer (1983) studied the functioning of patient care units in a teaching hospital. Their study provides some evidence about the effectiveness of different coordinating mechanisms in a health care setting. Modifying the March and Simon classification of coordinating activities, Charns and Schaefer described three different types of programmed coordination and three types of nonprogrammed coordination, as follows.

Types of Programmed Coordination

1. *Work process standardization* involves the use of rules, schedules, plans, and protocols.

2. *Skill standardization* entails education and on-the-job training to ensure that tasks are performed at a level exceeding some predetermined minimum level of competence.

3. *Output standardization* refers to the form or outcome of work as it moves through different stages. Workers at each new stage always receive the same output from workers in the previous stage.

Types of Nonprogrammed Coordination

1. *Supervision* is the exchange of information that occurs when one individual is clearly responsible for the work of another.

2. *Mutual adjustment* is the informal exchange of information about work performance between two individuals in the work group who are not responsible for each other's job performance.

3. *Group coordination* is the use of meetings involving more than two people to exchange information.

Nonprogrammed coordination is also known as *feedback coordination*. Charns and Schaefer observed that feedback methods of coordination are more time consuming but may be needed when there is a high degree of uncertainty about the work being performed. In their assessment of hospital patient care units, they found that high-performing units made greater use of all six methods of coordination and were more likely to use feedback methods in unfamiliar situations. Furthermore, work group members with less experience needed to use feedback methods of coordination to a greater extent than more experienced members. For feedback methods to be effective, work group members needed a considerable degree of trust and understanding, and these qualities were more likely to be present when the group's composition was consistent over time. Charns and Schaefer also concluded that, when a group did not fully achieve coordination, its performance was hampered. In that situation, work group members were likely to be frustrated because their hard work did not lead to the desired outcome.

In summary, this literature suggests that it is a significant challenge for members of a chronic illness management work group to coordinate tasks effectively. Different methods of coordination are likely to be required for various tasks and for different work group members. In some cases, extensive programmed and nonprogrammed efforts at coordination may be required. For instance, in the early stages of a chronic illness management work group's development, patients may not be skilled or experienced in carrying out their roles. They may require protocols to guide them (work process standardization) and considerable training (skill standardization). At the same time, because of their inexperience, they may require feedback through mutual adjustment or group coordination processes.

This need is consistent with a "coaching" style of leadership, as described above, and will require substantial time on the part of at least some group members. A member may need to assume a liaison role, accepting responsibility for the overall coordination of group activities, in order for the group to operate effectively. In clinical models of chronic illness management, this liaison role is frequently assumed by a nurse who is trained to be a chronic disease "specialist."

The Importance of Assessing Performance

Virtually all standard theories of management include the measurement of performance. Approaches based on management by objectives (MBO) stress the need to assess the performance of employees, groups, or organizational subunits continually by measuring their work against performance goals. Other approaches emphasize measuring performance against standards as a strategy for organizational control. Continuous Quality Improvement (CQI) programs redesign organizational processes based on performance data, with a particular emphasis on information gathered from customers.

These management models suggest the different reasons that assessing work group performance is typically an integral part of overall work group design. First, the work group is usually accountable to a larger organization. Assessing performance helps to establish the group's credibility within that organization; with increased confidence in the group, the organization will continue to support the work group's objectives by giving it necessary resources.

Second, groups need performance assessment so that they can respond to buyers who have concerns about the products they are purchasing. In health care, it is increasingly common for large employers, coalitions of employers, or public program administrators to purchase services through a formal proposal process. As part of this process, the health care organization receives a Request for Proposal (RFP), which often specifies how performance is to be measured and how performance information is to be conveyed to the purchaser. In response to this RFP, health care organizations or insurers submit bids. Thus, measuring work group performance is an integral part of the larger health care organization's efforts to respond to purchasers' demands for performance data.

Third, performance measurement is a necessary part of the intelligent redesign of structure and processes in organizations. In this context, work group members use performance data to assess what is going well and what is going poorly. They then implement changes to increase efficiency or improve product characteristics. The appeal of this aspect of performance measurement is reflected in the popularity of industrial models of quality improvement in the health care arena (Gottlieb, Margolis, and Schoenbaum, 1990), although the degree to which these models have been fully implemented at the work group level is sometimes questionable (Berwick, Baker, and Kramer, 1992).

Finally, the act of measuring performance has the inherent potential to improve performance. When work groups know they are being evaluated and have a clear understanding of the performance evaluation criteria, their performance may improve simply because members carry out their tasks more intelligently and energetically.

Just as there is substantial agreement that it is important to measure work group performance, there is also agreement that any evaluation process must address two key questions: What should be measured? How should it be measured? The answers to these questions will vary across work groups and the nature of the work they perform. The answers will also depend on the overall strategy for performance measurement adopted by the group's parent organization. In general, no single measure will satisfy all of the different demands for performance information. This raises the additional question of how the different measures should be weighted to assess the group's overall performance. Typically, both process and outcome measures are used to assess work group performance. For instance, with respect to a chronic illness management work group, a process measure might address the proportion of patients whose health status is assessed according to some predetermined schedule, whereas an outcome measure might address patients' satisfaction with their ability to manage some of the negative consequences associated with their illnesses. The choice of what to measure, and what weights to attach to multiple measures, is clearly important in a chronic illness management work group, because these values will motivate certain types of performance, add legitimacy to specific activities within the work group, and send signals to group members concerning organizational goals and objectives for the group.

The three features of chronic illness, as discussed above, have implications for designing appropriate performance assessment processes for chronic illness management work groups. For instance, chronic illness's longitudinal nature has significant bearing on the time frame used to assess performance. This is often an issue for performance measurement in health care, as Charns and Schaefer (1983) observe with respect to the assessment of acute care delivered in a hospital: "Effectiveness assessed over the short run may not relate to effectiveness over the long term. Sometimes what appears effective in the short run is actually a suboptimization when viewed over the longer term. . . . Another aspect of time as it relates to effectiveness is that some organizational outcomes are not known for very long periods of time, and thus a usable assessment is not feasible" (p. 47). These assessment issues clearly apply to chronic illness management work groups, as well. Pressures to demonstrate effectiveness in the short term can lead groups to adopt measures of outcomes without evidence that these measures are linked to patient satisfaction or improved functioning in the long term. It is particularly difficult to demonstrate improvement in patient outcomes without meaningful comparison groups that can be followed for long periods; given this deficit, assessment measures of outcomes have even less validity.

A second characteristic of chronic illnesses—the large number of individuals or even organizations involved in treating an individual patient—also has implications for performance assessment.

Charns and Schaefer (1983) note that "different people place different values on different outcomes. For example, a patient would evaluate the effectiveness of a hospital primarily in terms of the care it provided. An intern or resident, on the other hand, would place greatest weight on its educational aspects and its contribution to professional development. Thus, what is an effective organization from one perspective might not be from another perspective" (p. 47). The relatively large number of individuals with different roles involved in treating a chronic illness increases the likelihood that work group members will place different values on various outcomes. Employees of the health care organization may place greater weight on process or financial measures of performance that are of interest to organization administrators and that can be used to secure or maintain organizational support for the work group's activities. Patients, on the other hand, can be expected to place greater emphasis on their satisfaction with services or their success in managing the limitations associated with their conditions. The weights that a group ultimately attaches (either implicitly or explicitly) to various measures of work group performance can provide insight for health care organization managers into work group orientation.

The patient's central role in the chronic illness work group can also affect the assessment of work group performance. The literature on work groups suggests that group members' involvement in setting goals and developing performance measures is critical to the success of the evaluation process. This means that chronic illness management work groups should elicit goals and discuss performance measures with patients in the early stages of work group development. Chronically ill patients must understand and value the assessment process because many of the performance measures that the group adopts are likely to require the patient's active participation. For instance, data needed to construct measures of patient satisfaction and coping skills can be collected only from patients' surveys. If patients are not convinced of the relevance of collecting and assessing data on work group performance, then even the most elegant evaluation designs will be infeasible in practice. Patients must be involved not only in the management of their own illnesses but also in the overall assessment of the care process.

Implications for Improving Chronic Illness Management

A common theme that has arisen in this chapter's discussion of chronic illness management work groups is the need to design work groups and their activities to support patients and respond to their concerns. Chronic illness management work groups are likely to evolve through predictable stages that reflect, to a great degree, the stages of patient development as partners in the management of their chronic illness. Clinicians will need to adopt different styles of group participation to accommodate different stages of patient development if work groups are to be successful. Clinicians need to be educated in the dynamics of work group development and leadership skills. Furthermore, they must be prepared to use various different means of communication and coordination in order to secure and maintain effective patient involvement in the work group. The diverse nature of the participants in a chronic illness management work group suggests that a particular work group member (usually a specially trained nurse) will need to assume a defined liaison role.

Not only do patients need to be effective members of work groups in order for these groups to be successful but they also must be involved in decisions about assessing work group performance. Without their involvement, it is not likely that this important activity can be carried out successfully. Again, this is consistent with the emphasis on patient education and involvement in chronic illness management as reflected in the chronic illness team models described in Chapter Three.

6

Work Group Models in Action
Experiences of Ongoing Programs

In Chapters Three through Five, we drew on the published literature relating to chronic illness and its treatment, as well as the literature on work groups, to identify critical issues relating to the organization and delivery of care to persons with chronic illness. However, a great deal of important knowledge regarding chronic illness management is not captured in formal models and evaluations. There are many ongoing, innovative programs in chronic illness management that have not been evaluated in a formal sense. Or when evaluation results are available, they do not always describe how programs are structured and organized. As we noted in Chapter Three, these issues in general tend to receive very little attention in studies that focus on the clinical aspects of care delivery.

Through a review of the literature, including trade journals, we identified organizations that had implemented, or were in the process of implementing, innovative approaches to managing diabetes, asthma, or arthritis. Then, in late 1995, we conducted telephone interviews with program directors, researchers, and care coordinators who were involved with these programs. In this chapter, we describe eight ongoing chronic illness management efforts and emphasize how they function in practice. These efforts range from relatively small-scale initiatives aimed at caring more effectively for targeted groups of patients to major efforts to revamp care processes in large managed care organizations. The components of each initiative are listed in tables. Together, the program descriptions illustrate how chronic illness management initiatives are being implemented in real-world settings.

Geisinger Health Plan: Asthma Treatment Program

The Geisinger Health Plan in Danville, Pennsylvania, has developed a program for asthma patients with the goal of increasing patient adherence to medication and treatment plans. (See Table 6.1.) This initiative includes a patient education program based on the National Asthma Education and Preventive Program (NAEPP) guidelines. The program has been implemented at nine primary care sites in Pennsylvania that the plan administers. These sites primarily serve lower- to middle-class patients who live in rural areas.

A randomized trial is under way to test how the provision of free medications affects patient adherence to treatment plans, quality of care, and the use of acute care services. Patients randomly assigned to the free medication group can only receive the free medicine if they attend education sessions and meet minimum standards of asthma self-care knowledge and skills, as assessed through objective measurements. Control group members also take part in patient education sessions but do not receive free medication.

Each site employs a nurse to administer the program, act as care coordinator for patients, and provide feedback to primary care physicians. The nurse provides patient education and collects data for program evaluation. A nurse-coordinator oversees operations for the entire program, which a general internist leads. An evaluation will address quality-of-life issues, service use, cost, patient satisfaction, and clinician compliance to NAEPP guidelines. The study's results will be used to determine the feasibility of incorporating the program into ongoing clinical practice within the organization.

Table 6.1. Geisinger Health Plan: Asthma Treatment Program.

Victor Villagra, Medical Director

Organization	• Geisinger Health Plan, Danville, Pennsylvania.
Program	• *Number of participants:* Approximately 250.
	• *Duration of program:* Twenty-four months, beginning in January 1995.
	• *Goals:* To determine whether providing incentive (free medications and supplies) and education increases compliance, improves quality of care, and reduces need for acute care services, as compared with providing education alone.
Population Served	• All patients who are two years old and older (no upper age limit), who have been diagnosed with asthma, and who have been seen at one of the nine primary care clinics.
	• Rural population with low income and educational levels.
Referral Source	• The patient population is limited to those asthma patients seen at the plan's nine primary care sites.
Components of Model	• A randomized trial is under way to test the effect of free medicines.
	• All patients enter the Asthma Education Program.
	• Patients who are randomly assigned to a "free medication arm of the study" must earn fifty points between visits to receive medications and supplies at no cost. They earn points by following medication instructions, viewing videos, using peak-flow meters, completing daily diaries, and so forth.
Team Members	• *Nurse specialist:* Is site coordinator at each office; provides patient education and staff education, oversees data collection and staff education; interacts with primary care physicians.
	• *Nurse-coordinator:* Oversees all site coordinators; holds meetings twice a month for providing updates and sharing experiences.
	• *Pharmacist:* Coordinates distribution of free medication; tracks overall pharmacy utilization.
Program Evaluation	• Results of the study will be assessed to determine if the project will be continued as a clinical program.
	• Measures include quality of life, utilization, cost, patient satisfaction, compliance with NAEPP guidelines.
Education for	• The pulmonologist and program director give all primary care physicians education on asthma and
Primary Care Physicians	NAE guidelines; follow-up education is available as needed.
Financial Issues	• Patients who are randomly selected receive free medications and supplies, whereas the other patients pay for medications and supplies according to health plan policies.
	• The ongoing program may be expanded to fifty-four clinics and presented to other payers (such as Blue Cross/Blue Shield) as a reimbursable program, if warranted by the research findings.

Source: Institute for Research and Education.

Harvard Pilgrim Health Care: Pediatric Asthma Program

Begun in 1993, the Central Pediatric Asthma Program (CPAP) at Harvard Pilgrim Health Care in Massachusetts seeks to improve patient self-management skills and medication compliance and to support primary care physicians in providing care that conforms with the guidelines for the diagnosis and management of asthma from the Expert Panel Report (National Asthma Education and Preventive Program). (See Table 6.2.) The program reaches children at fourteen inner-city, urban, and suburban HMO practice settings. Children qualify for participation in the CPAP if an exacerbation of their asthma has prompted a recent emergency room visit or hospitalization or if their primary care physician refers them to the program. Program evaluation is ongoing and includes monitoring the utilization of services.

Five outreach pediatric nurses with extensive training in asthma are each assigned to three to four centers and are responsible for identifying moderate- to high-risk asthmatics who would benefit from the program. Once the patient is identified and enrolled in the program, the outreach nurse meets with the patient and family members to assess the severity of the disease and to design an individualized disease management program. The nurse provides one-on-one education for patients and family members, focusing on their knowledge of the condition, triggers, early warning signs, environmental issues, and self-management skills. The nurse makes follow-up phone calls in response to the patient's needs. The program also includes a multidisciplinary team review of difficult cases, in which the director (a pediatrician specializing in asthma), an allergist, a psychiatrist, and the patient's primary care physician all give input. The primary care physician provides ongoing medical care.

Table 6.2. Harvard Pilgrim Health Care: Central Pediatric Asthma Program.

Kathleen Loane, Outreach Asthma Nurse, Clinical Coordinator
Walter Torda, Director

Organization	• Harvard Pilgrim Health Care—Health Center Division, Boston, Massachusetts.
Program	• *Number of participants:* Approximately five hundred as of summer 1996. • *Duration of program:* Began in November 1993. • *Goals:* (1) To improve patient and family compliance with treatment recommendations, (2) to improve patient and family self-management skills, (3) to decrease variability of care and increase conformity with guidelines from the Expert Panel Report (NAEPP), (4) to support primary care teams caring for children with asthma.
Population Served	• Children up to eighteen years old who receive care through the Health Center Division (fourteen health centers in inner-city, urban, and suburban settings). • Patients identified via (1) ER visit or hospitalization, (2) referral by primary care physician, and (3) Medicaid monthly enrollment list identifying individuals with asthma. High risk criteria for automatic enrollment include hospitalization of a child less than five years of age; two or more hospitalizations in a lifetime; hospital stay of three or more days' duration; a life-threatening case of asthma (for example, severity of asthma requiring ICU admission or intubation); or poor functional status.
Referral Source	• Primary care physicians and outreach nurses.
Components of Model	• An outreach nurse is assigned to three to four health centers and is responsible for identifying patients who are moderate- to high-risk asthmatics via daily monitoring of hospital or ER utilization. • Additional referrals are obtained from primary care physicians. • Multidisciplinary team 1. The nurse meets the patient and family for an in-depth interview about asthma. The patient may only need to see the outreach nurse for education and follow-up support. The patient then continues follow-up asthma care with the primary care physician only.

Table 6.2. Harvard Pilgrim Health Care: Central Pediatric Asthma Program, *continued.*

2. If ideal results are not reached, despite the involvement of the pediatrician and asthma outreach nurse, the case is presented at the program's monthly central multidisciplinary team meeting. The team makes recommendations to the child's pediatrician.

3. If the patient's asthma continues to remain poorly controlled, a personal, multifocal evaluation with the specialist is arranged. Clinical sessions with specialists are available on a weekly basis.

- The nurse's role includes one-on-one education with the patient and family, which may require one to three visits in which information is provided on asthma, triggers, early warning signs, medications, equipment, and environmental control. Follow-up calls are scheduled as frequently as necessary for each patient.

- The nurse also identifies barriers that prevent control of asthma, including access to health care, lack of knowledge regarding the disease or use of the health care system, and psychosocial issues.

Team Members	- *Outreach nurse with pediatric background and extensive training in asthma:* Define the need for case management; provide education; monitor patient progress.
	- *Allergist:* Provides consultation; attends CPAP meetings.
	- *Primary care physician.*
	- *Pediatrician:* Is medical director of the program; specializes in asthma.
	- *Psychiatrist:* Provides expertise in addressing family and patient mental health issues; is available for patient consultation as needed.
	- *Patient and family:* Apply self-management techniques learned in the program.
Program Evaluation	- An ongoing evaluation examines data on utilization, satisfaction, and patient's functional status.
Education for Primary Care Physicians	- There is a mandatory four-hour continuing medication education class for primary care physicians regarding NIH guidelines, plus a follow-up session (1.5 hours).
Financial Issues	- The inner-city patient population with Medicaid or health plan coverage has free prescriptions.
	- The working inner-city population that is non-Medicaid either has a copayment for medications or has no drug plan.

Source: Institute for Research and Education.

Rush Prudential Health Plans: Pediatric Asthma Nurse Care Management Program

The Rush Prudential HMO in Chicago has implemented a specialized disease management program for children with asthma and their families (Zablocki, 1995). Staff nurses and physicians teach biannual asthma education classes. These two-hour group classes address topics such as how the lungs function, how to recognize subjective signs and symptoms of an asthma attack, how medications work, and how to use peak-flow meters. (See Table 6.3.)

In addition to giving these education sessions, Rush Prudential is currently piloting an extensive management program for children with severe asthma who have experienced multiple emergency room visits or hospitalizations. These patients receive a two-hour multidimensional assessment conducted by the nurse case manager and reviewed by the team. The team includes pediatricians and pediatric allergists, a psychologist, the patient's primary care physician, and a nurse case manager. Following this assessment, the team forms a treatment plan that focuses on weaknesses in the patient's self-management and methods for improvement. The plan is then shared with the patient and family.

The treatment plan includes an intensive phase, an intermediate phase, a transition phase, and an independent phase. During the intensive phase, the case manager calls the patient or family every three to seven days to monitor the patient, check compliance, continue teaching, and review the treatment plan if necessary. During the intermediate phase, the case manager calls every fourteen days for the same purposes. During the transition phase, calls occur just once a month. In the independent phase, the case manager does not call the patient or family but is available to answer questions. If children are admitted to the hospital because of asthma at any time during this intensive program, they must begin again with the intensive phase. A program evaluation will include a cost-effectiveness analysis, a review of patient satisfaction, and an assessment of patient outcomes.

Table 6.3. Rush Prudential Health Plans: Pediatric Asthma Nurse Case Management Program.

Mary Pat Paquette, Pediatric Asthma Nurse

Organizations	• Rush Prudential Health Plans (a prepaid mixed-model HMO plan, one of three products offered by RPHP), Chicago, Illinois. • Center for Health Services Research and Nursing Services Research and Support, Rush Presbyterian St. Luke's Medical Center—Chicago, Illinois.
Program	Pediatric Asthma Nurse Case Management Pilot Program. • *Number of participants:* Forty children with asthma identified as high risk (two or more hospitalizations in a year; three or more ER visits in a year; two or more ER visits plus one hospitalization in a year; or one hospitalization of more than five days). • *Duration of program:* The program began in May 1995. • *Goals:* To determine whether a nurse case management program for children with asthma will improve patient symptoms, functional status, and satisfaction; will decrease ER and hospital use; and will be cost effective.
Population Served	• Children through age eighteen with asthma who are seen at HMO offices. The population served is multicultural with varying education and income levels.
Referral Source	• Review of utilization and claims data.
Components of Model	All participants receive a full initial assessment. Half then are randomly assigned to a multidisciplinary team approach, and half receive customary care. • *Initial assessment:* Two-hour interview done by case manager (CM) at an appointment that two other family or caregivers can attend. This interview uses a 300-question assessment tool and caregiver questionnaire assessing quality of life, caregiver stress, functional status, environmental allergens, and so forth. Children nine years and older have a separate interview assessing medication responsibility and compliance and inhaler and peak-flow technique. • *Multidisciplinary team meetings:* The CM and the primary care physician present the results of the initial assessment to the team. The team discusses issues and barriers to wellness, determines risk factors for nine domains (asthma knowledge, medication adherence, self-management, family dynamics, and so on), and develops a treatment plan. • *Clinical meetings:* The CM and head of pediatrics meet weekly, or as needed, to discuss clinical issues. • *Four-phase program:* (The time frame for each phase varies, depending on the needs of the patient and family.) *Intensive phase* (approximately three months): The patient (and family) meets with the CM weekly to address high-risk domains or issues. The CM calls every 3–7 days to reinforce and support the patient and family.

Intermediate phase (approximately three months): The patient (and family) meets with the CM every two to three weeks. The CM calls every fourteen days to reinforce and support the patient.

Transition phase (approximately three months): The patient (and family) meets with the CM every four to five weeks for support. The CM calls once a month to provide support.

Independent phase (approximately six to eight months): The patient (and family) are proficient in self-management and initiate contact with the CM as needed. If the patient has an ER visit or hospitalization for asthma, this is considered a treatment failure and the patient reenters the program at the intensive phase.

Team Members
- *Head of Pediatrics.*
- *Pediatric asthma nurse:* Makes initial assessment; provides ongoing phone monitoring; maintains communication with primary care physician and specialists.
- *Primary care physician:* Conducts ongoing case review with CM; can call for team review if patient status changes.
- *Psychologist:* Is a resource for the team; is available to see patient and family as needed.
- *Pediatric allergist:* Is a resource for the team; sees patients as needed.
- *Research team* from Nursing Services Research and Support and the Center for Health Services Research at Rush Presbyterian St. Luke's Medical Center: Actively assesses program, protocol, and tools and identifies need for changes.

Program Evaluation
- *Principal outcomes:* Symptom-free days.
- *Secondary analysis:* Utilization (ER visits, hospitalizations), functional status, satisfaction with program, and so forth.
- *Additional analysis:* Cost-effectiveness (dollars spent, symptom-free days gained) and cost-benefit (dollars spent, dollars saved in utilization).
- *Process evaluation:* Examination of types and intensities of interventions.

Education for Primary Care Physicians
- Physicians learn techniques to treat and manage asthma as part of the pilot project team; NIH guidelines are distributed to all pediatricians.
- Allergists give mandatory in-service training on guidelines.
- The CM is a resource for primary care physicians on an ongoing basis and provides in-service training to office nurses about peak-flow meters.

Financial Issues
- The pilot is internally funded by three organizations.
- Discussions are under way regarding funding for ongoing programs. It is anticipated that the nurse case management program will be a free service to patients.

Source: Institute for Research and Education.

Columbia Hospital: Arthritis Treatment Center

The Columbia Musculoskeletal Institute at Columbia Hospital in Milwaukee, Wisconsin, hosts the Arthritis Day Treatment Program at Columbia Arthritis Center. (See Table 6.4.) The program, which began in 1983, provides comprehensive treatment and education in an outpatient setting for adults with various rheumatic diseases.

Rheumatologists from the Columbia Musculoskeletal Institute refer most patients to the program. Patients complete preassessment surveys that are specific to particular rheumatic conditions. The referring physician conducts a medical assessment and writes orders for the patient to participate in the Arthritis Day Treatment Program.

When the program begins, an arthritis nurse-coordinator provides a four- to six-hour session, giving one-on-one patient and family education about the disease and self-management skills and addressing psychosocial issues. Based on the patient's individual needs, the nurse can order other specialty services, such as nutritional counseling from a dietitian and physical or occupational therapy. Patients with complex needs return to the center to complete the initial program and to have their progress reviewed a month later. The referring physician receives a summary of the assessment and care plan.

New outreach initiatives are under way that use the skills of the arthritis nurse-coordinator even further. These nurse-led programs include free arthritis screening for patients at a rural outpatient therapy facility and demonstrations of arthritis-screening techniques for medical students at a local family practice clinic.

Currently, a program evaluation focuses on patient satisfaction with the program. Previous evaluations have addressed physician satisfaction and financial issues. These evaluations suggested that physicians were very satisfied with the services provided, felt that the program was needed, and thought it supplemented usual patient care.

Table 6.4. Columbia Hospital: Columbia Arthritis Center.

Janice Smith Pigg, Former Director, Consultant

Organization	• Columbia Arthritis Center, Columbia Musculoskeletal Institute, Columbia Hospital, Milwaukee, Wisconsin.
Program	• Arthritis Day Treatment Program.
	• *Number of participants*: One to three patients per day.
	• *Duration of program*: Started in 1983.
	• *Goals*: To maintain comprehensive treatment and educational programming for ambulatory rheumatic disease patients (previously seen in an inpatient setting).
Population Served	• Mainly adults with arthritis.
Referral Source	• Most referrals come directly from rheumatologists, but some come from primary care physicians.
	• For patients who call without a physician referral, the program staff contacts the patient's physician with information on the program and a request for approval.
Components of Model	• Preliminary screening is done by the physician who refers to the Arthritis Day Treatment Program.
	• There is a detailed preassessment via patient survey that is specific to arthritis, osteoporosis, or fibromyalgia.
	• An individualized program is developed that includes therapy, nutrition, patient education in a one-on-one four-to six-hour session, and a medical assessment by a rheumatologist. Family participation is encouraged.
	• The rheumatologist sends a summary and care plan to the primary care physician.
Team Members	• *Rheumatologist or primary care physician*: Does the preliminary assessment; refers to a day treatment program; writes orders for a treatment plan.
	• *Nurse-coordinator, case manager*: Provides education, social services; addresses mental health issues; calls in other professionals as needed, such as mental health, orthotist, and pedorthist. Augments the rheumatologist's orders for treatment according to patient need, and informs physicians of changes.
	• *Dietitian*: Provides nutritional assessment and patient education.
	• *Physical therapist and occupational therapist*: Provides exercise programs, stress management, and adaptive equipment.

Table 6.4. Columbia Hospital: Columbia Arthritis Center, *continued*.

Program Evaluation	• The present evaluation focuses on patient satisfaction. Previously evaluations have addressed financial viability and physician satisfaction.
Ongoing Program for Patients	• Complex patients come back for follow-up visit within a month.
	• Two additional programs are under way: (1) free arthritis screening by a nurse or case manager at a rural outpatient therapy facility, and (2) arthritis screening by a nurse at a family practice center (training ground for residents).
Education for Primary Care Physicians	• An annual summer conference on a rheumatology topic is geared to the primary care physician and recently has been shortened from one day to two hours.
Financial Issues	• This multidisciplinary program is now changing, because of cutbacks in funding and other reimbursement issues (Medicare regulations, capitation, and so forth). Some patient populations now are being seen in a sporadic fashion, again because of changes in reimbursement.

Source: Institute for Research and Education.

St. Elizabeth Hospital:
Arthritis Treatment Center

The Arthritis Treatment Center is a program of the St. Elizabeth Hospital Rehabilitation Center located at the LaSalle Clinic in Menasha, Wisconsin. (See Table 6.5.) This program is designed for patients of all ages with any form of arthritis, and it serves both HMO and fee-for-service patients from northeast Wisconsin and Michigan. Similar to other team care models, the program includes a rheumatologist, an arthritis nurse-coordinator who serves as a care manager, an occupational therapist, a physical therapist, and other rehabilitation specialists who are called on as needed.

Referrals to the program come from rheumatologists at the LaSalle Clinic and from local primary care practitioners and rheumatologists. Patients who have been referred to the center meet first with team members to devise a care plan. An educational program to teach patients self-care and self-management techniques is provided within the first three months of enrollment. A follow-up program is available once a patient has demonstrated a firm grasp of self-management techniques.

The team convenes once a month to discuss new cases and review the progress of care for continuing patients. The rheumatologists monitor ongoing treatment and medications and maintain contact with the referring physician through periodic status reports.

An assessment of program effectiveness is being conducted. Outcome measures will include patient satisfaction and functional status.

Group Health Cooperative of Puget Sound:
Diabetes Mini-Clinics

Group Health Cooperative in Seattle, Washington, is conducting a randomized controlled trial to test the feasibility of a chronic care model for diabetes patients. (See Table 6.6.) The model includes mini-clinics held at primary care sites at regular intervals.

Table 6.5. St. Elizabeth Hospital: Arthritis Treatment Center.

Karen Meyer, Nurse-Coordinator

Organization	• The Arthritis Treatment Center is a specialty program of the St. Elizabeth Hospital Rehabilitation Center located at the LaSalle Clinic (a clinic with a neuromusculoskeletal focus), Menasha, Wisconsin.
Program	• *Number of participants:* About two hundred of the four hundred or more referrals in 1995 received coordinated services at the center.
	• *Duration of program:* The Arthritis Treatment Center was developed in 1988.
	• *Goals:* To provide comprehensive, coordinated, interdisciplinary team evaluation and treatment services that are designed to help people of all ages with rheumatologic conditions achieve or maintain a functional level consistent with a productive and independent lifestyle.
Population Served	• People of all ages with rheumatic diseases in northeast Wisconsin and Upper Michigan.
Referral Source	• LaSalle Clinic rheumatologists refer 98 percent of treatment center patients.
Components of Model	• Arthritis Treatment Center is an outpatient program with a team approach.
	• Initial evaluation is done by the rheumatologist, who refers patient to the team; after the team completes its evaluations, the care plan is discussed at team meetings.
	The team meets every two to four weeks to discuss new referrals and review active cases.
	• On average, it takes about three months after the initial evaluation to complete treatment, provide education, and establish a self-managed program.
	• Follow-up visits occur at three, six, nine, and twelve months, depending on patient needs, which are determined after the patient has a good grasp of self-management concepts.
	• Medical monitoring and the monitoring of medications, lab results, and so on, is done by LaSalle Clinic rheumatologists; these activities are not part of this specific model.

Team Members	• *Rheumatologist*: Refers patients that meet the Arthritis Treatment Center admission criteria and directs their overall treatment. • *Rheumatology nurse-coordinator*: Responsible for patient case management; coordination of services; program administration; patient and family education about the disease process, self-management strategies, coping skills, lifestyle changes, medications, and so forth. • *Occupational and physical therapists*: Assess the patient's overall functional status, develop exercise programs, and provide assistive devices. • *Team members*: Refer to other rehabilitation professionals and specialists as appropriate (for example, biofeedback, psychology or psychiatry, dietitian); for more complex cases, insurance CMs also join team meetings and educational sessions with patients.
Program Evaluation	• A patient satisfaction survey is sent upon discharge from the program. • In the past, the Arthritis Impact Measurement Scale Fibromyalgia Impact Questionnaire, and Knowledge Questionnaire have been used. • Outcomes measures are being reexamined.
Education for Primary Care Physicians	• Area hospitals offer monthly educational presentations on medical issues. • Rheumatologists participate in rheumatological presentations about once a year for the hospital's medical staff.
Financial Issues	• All services are fee-for-service. • Recently, a case management charge was added to cover team meetings and case management.

Source: Institute for Research and Education.

Table 6.6. Group Health Cooperative of Puget Sound: Diabetes Mini-Clinics.

Michael Von Korff, Associate Director

Organization	• Group Health Cooperative of Puget Sound, Seattle, Washington.
Program	Diabetes and Frail Elderly Mini-Clinics • *Number of participants:* Approximately eight hundred. • *Duration of program:* Pilot, 1992; Randomized trial, 1994–1996. • *Goals:* To develop a chronic care clinic model; to implement the model throughout the central region of Group Health's service area; to assess whether the innovation produces increased compliance with guidelines for care, improvements in adherence with self-management behaviors, improvements in clinical status and quality of life, reductions in hospital and emergency room use and health care costs, and improvements in patient and primary care provider satisfaction.
Population Served	• Diabetes patients of all ages who are seen by Group Health primary care physicians.
Referral Source	• Patients are identified for the program via a diabetes registry at Group Health. • Patients will eventually be able to self-refer to the mini-clinics.
Components of Model	• The program supports primary care physicians. It includes a mini-clinic for diabetics tailored around their specific needs through ancillary services. • The initial mini-clinic visit is three to four hours, including one-on-one visits for patients with various team members and ending with a group session led by a social worker. • Follow-up visits are one to two hours, with their need defined by the primary care physician. The follow-up visit also includes group sessions (with the same group of patients that participated in the group session at the initial visit).
Team Members	• *Primary care physician:* Provides clinical assessment and ongoing care. • *Primary care nurse:* Has one-on-one appointment with patient for routine assessment and education about self-management. • *Pharmacist:* Consults about medication management.

- *Nutritionist*: Does one-on-one nutrition consultation.
- *Social Worker*: Provides one-on-one psychosocial support; leads patient group sessions.
- *Diabetologist and diabetic nurse specialist*: Are available to provide consultation as needed to the primary care team on site.

Program Evaluation	The program is being evaluated using a randomized controlled trial. Program evaluation includes a patient survey (functional status, satisfaction, improvement of self-management behaviors); a survey to assess provider satisfaction; and an assessment of the program's impact on utilization (that is, on decrease in hospitalizations and ER use).
Education for Primary Care Physicians	A nurse-educator provides population-based management training, which is required of all physicians and nurses. It includes use of guidelines for health care delivery.
Financial Issues	Payment for program components is through the HMO's health care coverage. A single copayment is required for the mini-clinic visit. This copayment applies to ancillary services, as well. Minimal replacement dollars are allocated to health care teams for clinic coordination.

Source: Institute for Research and Education.

These clinics are staffed by a multispecialty team, including a diabetologist, a diabetic nurse specialist, a nutritionist, a social worker, and a pharmacist. Under the mini-clinic model, the primary care physician and nurse maintain responsibility for the clinical assessment and ongoing care of patients. They provide patient education on self-management behaviors. This physician and nurse consult with the diabetologist, diabetes nurse specialist, and other mini-clinic team members and seek their support as needed.

This model was developed to support primary care physicians and to provide care tailored to the needs of each diabetic patient. Training programs about the patient's care and about the use of guidelines for health care delivery are provided for all primary care physicians and nurses.

Initial mini-clinic visits are three to four hours long and include one-on-one visits with various team members and a group session led by a social worker. Follow-up visits are shorter and include group sessions.

Evaluation of the mini-clinics will assess clinician compliance with guidelines, and will include surveys to measure the patient's functional status, satisfaction with care, and self-management skills. Provider satisfaction and the program's impact on utilization will also be measured.

Kaiser Permanente of Northern California: Diabetes Model

Kaiser Permanente of Northern California, a group-model HMO with 2.4 million members, is currently designing, implementing, and evaluating new models of integrated care for patients with chronic illnesses. (See Table 6.7.) Ongoing evaluation of these new models of care will provide the organization with information about patient outcomes and cost effectiveness. If appropriate, the evaluation findings will be used to promote organizationwide implementation of changes in processes of care for these patients.

Table 6.7. Kaiser Permanente, Northern California: Diabetes Model.

Joe Selby, Assistant Director

Organization	• Kaiser Permanente, Northern California, is a group-model HMO with 2.4 million members.
	• Services are delivered through fifteen hospital-based medical centers and seventeen freestanding medical office buildings.
	• The regional offices dedicated to health education, quality and utilization, and research work together with the Regional New Models of Care Committee to design, implement, and evaluate new models of integrated care for chronic illnesses.
Program	• A New Model of Care for Diabetes.
	• A Regional Diabetes Task Force was charged with developing a new model of intensive care for diabetics (both type I and type II).
	• Three alternative approaches to intensive primary care have been described: (1) nurse case management, (2) cluster visits, and (3) multidisciplinary clinics.
	• All feature increased reliance on nonphysicians (that is, nurses, nurse-educators) but are organized differently.
	• The cost of care for treating diabetes and its complications was calculated and a cost-effectiveness model is being built to help guide allocation of resources.
	• An internally funded, randomized trial of cluster visits (compared with usual care) began in July 1995. It involves six hundred adult patients over an eighteen-month period. Trials of nurse case management are in the planning phase.
	• Goals: (1) To improve both short-term clinical outcomes (hemoglobin A_{1C} levels, ketoacidosis rates) and long-term outcomes (micro- and macrovascular complication rates), (2) to improve satisfaction of patients and providers, (3) to improve performance of prevention measures, and (4) to achieve cost neutrality within two years.
Population Served	• There are 85,209 health plan members with diabetes mellitus primarily in the San Francisco and Sacramento areas.
Referral Source	• A diabetes registry identifies all patients with diabetes.
	• A key question will be how to target the new model's more intensive services to members most likely to benefit.
Components of Model	• "Near real-time" diabetes registry: Identifies patients with diabetes via pharmacy data, abnormal hemoglobin A_{1C} or hospital discharge. The registry is updated every six months. The intent is to make the system real-time and incorporate it into clinical practice.

Table 6.7. Kaiser Permanente, Northern California: Diabetes Model, *continued*.

- *Patient-tracking system*: Uses the registry as a "tickler system" to identify patients at high risk, patients who need an eye exam, and so on.
- *Evidence-based care guidelines*: Process begun to identify clinicians willing to be on a team that will develop guidelines.
- *Targeted use of nurse case management*: Has just begun. The hope is to determine cost-effectiveness of using nonphysician staff, such as diabetic nurse specialists who act as case managers.
- *Cluster visits*: Approximately twelve to twenty patients come together for group visits to provide health education and address psychosocial issues through a support group led by a nurse case manager and specialist. Appointments for eye care, foot care, and mental health care for individual patients is also available as needed during the group visit.
- *Increased use of peer support groups.*
- *Outcomes monitoring*: Review admission rates at fifteen hospitals and review hemoglobin A_{1C} levels.

Team Members	Direct patient care (cluster visits, nurse case management, multidisciplinary clinics)

- *Patient and family.*
- *Primary care physicians*: Manage overall care, with minimal involvement on the disease-specific team.
- *Nurse-educator case managers.*
- *Health educator*: Provides support to the team and is available for patient referrals.

Organizational system support
- *Regional Diabetes Task Force*: Is charged with developing a new model of intensive care for diabetics (both type I and type II).
- *Regional information service*: Maintains and customizes a tracking system.
- *Regional health education*: Supports nurse-educators at facilities.
- *Regional quality and utilization*: Develops diabetes care guidelines and monitors outcomes.
- *Regional research*: Evaluates specific components of new models of care (pilot studies) and validates new outcome measures.

Program Evaluation	• Randomized trial evaluations of the components of each new model are being planned or conducted. • There is ongoing monitoring of outcomes using automated databases (program effectiveness, patient satisfaction, functional assessment). • There is ongoing assessment of cost-effectiveness.
Education for Primary Care Physicians	• Education will begin when the care guidelines are finalized.
Financial Issues	• Neither anticipated costs nor expected benefits of the program are finalized. • Management would like new programs to be "cost-neutral" in a short time frame. • The costs of current care have been estimated. • A cost-effectiveness model is being developed, but having limited data on program effectiveness makes it difficult to estimate benefits.

Source: Institute for Research and Education.

One of the organization's initiatives in this area involves developing and testing three models of primary care delivery for diabetics. These approaches feature the increased use of nonphysician resources in managing diabetes. An established diabetes registry identifies and tracks patients at risk for diabetes, and it maintains information on pharmacy, laboratory, and hospitalization data for patients who have been diagnosed with diabetes.

The first model is a nurse case management program. Nurse case managers will coordinate care for diabetic patients, ensuring that they receive preventive services. Through the use of established processes, the nurse case manager will provide ongoing diabetes management for these patients, thus relieving primary care physicians of routine patient-monitoring activities.

A second care model was implemented in July 1995 as an eighteen-month randomized trial that compared "cluster visits" with usual care. In the cluster visits model, a group of twelve to twenty diabetic patients met at regular intervals for clinic appointments and peer support. They received health education and psychosocial support in group sessions led by a nurse specialist.

A third initiative is aimed specifically at type I diabetes. In this model, a multidisciplinary team of physician specialists, nurses, and social workers convenes in clinics to offer patients access to a variety of resources at one location.

Stanford University School of Medicine: Program for Management of Chronic Diseases

A Stanford University School of Medicine program for managing chronic diseases was implemented in the school's primary care services in late fall 1997. (See Table 6.8.) In the four-year experimental design, patients are randomly assigned to the new model of care management or to usual care at other health care sites.

The program educates patients about self-management techniques. Patient input is used in the design, implementation, and

Table 6.8. Stanford University School of Medicine: Program for Management of Chronic Diseases.

Halsted Holman, Director

Organization	• Stanford Primary Care Practices in Family Medicine and General Internal Medicine, Stanford University School of Medicine, Palo Alto, California.
Program	Program for Management of Chronic Diseases (PMCD).
	• All patients with chronic diseases will be affected by the program. A randomly selected one thousand individuals with chronic lung disease, arthritis, heart disease, diabetes, and lower back pain will experience the full intervention and the detailed outcome assessments.
	• The experimental program will last four years and began in fall 1997.
	• *Goals:* To improve the effectiveness and efficiency of health care and the satisfaction of patients and health professionals, through (1) training patients in skills for self-management and for partnership relations with health professionals; (2) training physicians and other health professionals to understand patients' perceptions of chronic illness, to facilitate and supervise patients' self-management activities, to create an effective partnership with patients and families, to eliminate conventional but unnecessary medical practices, and to engage in a variety of techniques for remote monitoring of patients as a substitute for office visits; (3) to train specialists to aid primary care physicians in the management of chronic disease; (4) to create a service infrastructure that facilitates the aforementioned goals; and (5) to involve students and residents in the new mechanisms of clinical practice.
Population Served	• All patients with chronic diseases receiving medical care by the primary care services.
Referral Source	• Stanford primary care physicians.
Components	• Patient education, especially for self-management.
	• Telephone management.
	• Home care, hospice care, remote monitoring, and mobile units.
	• Physician "firms," in which the same specialists work continuously with groups of primary care physicians.
	• Patient participation in the design, direction, and evaluation of health care services.

Table 6.8. Stanford University School of Medicine: Program for Management of Chronic Diseases, *continued*.

Team Members	• Primary care physicians. • Nurse practitioners and physician assistants. • Nurses and infrastructure staff. • Patients and families. • Specialists participating in firms. • Home care and hospice personnel.
Program Evaluation	• Evaluation will occur primarily by a self-administered questionnaire supplemented by information from the medical record and the institutional database, plus qualitative inquiry with selected subgroups of participants. • The evaluation will assess patient knowledge and behaviors, changes in health status, service utilization rates, patient and professional satisfaction, and program costs. • Evaluation data from randomized participants will be compared with similar data from comparison groups at other health care sites.
Education for Primary Care Physicians	Education will focus on improving primary care physicians' understanding of the following: • The importance of patient perceptions • The value of patient self-management and partnership relations between patients and physicians • Skills in supervising self-management and creating partnerships • Efficiency in deploying medical practices • Collaboration with specialists and uses of evaluation data
Financial Issues	• If successful, this program will save more resources than it expends, creating a potential model that can be applied in other settings.

Source: Institute for Research and Education.

evaluation of this new health care service. The program includes nurse practitioners and physician assistants who monitor patients by phone so that they need not visit the clinic. To provide a complete menu of care options for the patient, the program offers home care services and mobile units. In this model, physician education emphasizes the importance of patient perceptions, the development of partnerships between patients and physicians, and the integration of specialists with primary care physicians in treating patients.

Program evaluation will be based on patient questionnaires, along with information abstracted from patients' medical records and institutional databases. Evaluations will assess patient knowledge, adherence to management strategies, health status, satisfaction, and utilization of services, as well as program cost effectiveness.

Implications for Improving Chronic Illness Management

The programs described in this chapter share several components. They emphasize patient education, feature a prominent role for a nurse-coordinator, and evaluate (or plan to evaluate) a wide range of program outcomes.

Several programs identify issues relating to maintaining ongoing program funding. The programs are located in, or supported by, a variety of organizations, ranging from a medium-sized hospital to a very large health plan. This underscores the pervasiveness of health care organizations' interest in rethinking chronic illness management, as well as the general agreement across different types of organizations about some of the essential components of promising models.

Nevertheless, there are also significant differences across these models—differences that suggest fundamental questions in the design and implementation of new chronic illness treatment approaches. For instance, should these programs be integrated with primary practice or located in separate units? Can stable sources of ongoing financial support be found for these programs? There are likely to be a variety of appropriate answers to these questions because chronic illness programs exist in a variety of different organizational and community environments.

7

Design and Implementation
Principles in Chronic Illness
Management Programs

To discuss issues in the design and operation of chronic illness management programs, we convened a panel of experts. For each program described in Chapter Six, there was one representative, as well as the founder of the International Diabetes Center at HealthSystem Minnesota. The panel participated in an intensive one-day meeting, with the goal of developing a set of principles for successful chronic illness management programs. A portion of the meeting was devoted to discussion among the participants, focusing on different aspects of chronic illness management. (See Table 7.1 for a summary of each individual's background and responsibilities relating to chronic illness management.)

At the end of the meeting, participants were asked to propose basic principles for chronic illness management that reflected the tenor of the group's discussion. In this chapter, we present the panel's principles and related comments by members that illustrate these principles. These comments occurred at various points during the meeting; we have edited them and regrouped them under the principle they address. What we lose of the discussion's give-and-take in doing this, we gain in clarity.

As an overall goal, the panel agreed that "a successful chronic illness management program should, over time, be simultaneously effective, efficient, and satisfying to patients, families, providers, organizations, and the community. To be successful, a program must

Table 7.1. Expert Panel on Chronic Illness Management.

Donnell D. Etzwiler is president, founder and former chief medical officer of the International Diabetes Center in Minneapolis. He is recognized internationally as a leader in diabetes education and patient care. He is the past president of the American Diabetes Association, past vice president of the International Diabetes Federation, and codirector of the World Health Organization's Diabetes Collaborating Center for Diabetes Education and Computer Technology. Etzwiler was principal investigator of the National Institutes of Health's Diabetes Control and Complications Trial (DCCT). He is a senior member of the Institute of Medicine, serves on many national and international boards, and is a clinical professor at the University of Minnesota's Departments of Pediatrics and Family Practice and Community Medicine.

Halsted R. Holman is the director of the Stanford Arthritis Center and cochief, Division of Family and Community Medicine, at Stanford University School of Medicine. He was a consultant for Kaiser Permanente's Medical Group Ambulatory Practice Model Project and is a member of the advisory committee for Kaiser's Project on Chronic Care Coordination. His past role in developing and directing an innovative model of care for the management of chronic illness at Midpeninsula Health Service in the 1970s was the origin of his current work at Stanford. Holman and others are presently completing a design of a Program for Management of Chronic Disease to be installed in the Stanford Primary Care Practices.

Kathleen C. Loane has specialized in the field of allergy and asthma for ten years at Harvard Pilgrim Health Care (HPHC). She developed an innovative program for high-risk asthmatics, decreasing hospitalizations and emergency room utilization (*Archives of Pediatric and Adolescent Medicine*, 1995, vol. 149). She is currently the clinical coordinator of the Central Pediatric Asthma Program at HPHC, an active participant with the Asthma Improvement Network of Massachusetts, and a member of the Institute for Health Care Improvements Asthma Breakthrough Series.

Karen R. Meyer is the coordinator for the northeastern Wisconsin Arthritis Treatment Center. She has extensive experience in both rehabilitation nursing and utilization review. In her current role, Meyer is responsible for the case management and coordination of services for persons referred to the center, providing education for patients and family with an emphasis on self-management, collaboration with team members on treatment and discharge plans, and program development. In addition, as part of a nurse–social worker team in the Geriatric Assessment Clinic, Meyer has expertise in case management, program coordination, and development.

Mary Pat Paquette is the pediatric asthma nurse case manager for Rush Prudential Partners, a product of Rush Prudential HMO in Chicago. She has been a pediatric nurse for fourteen years with inpatient and ambulatory experience. She has written an asthma education book that Rush Prudential HMO uses and has coordinated and taught asthma education classes for patients and their parents or caregivers. Recently, she has participated in developing and implementing a clinical pediatric asthma case management program.

Janice Smith Pigg's clinical background is in rheumatology nursing. She is the primary author of *Rheumatology Nursing: A Problem Oriented Approach* (Pigg, Driscoll, and Caniff, 1985) and was cochair of the task force writing *Outcome Standards for Rheumatology Nursing Practice* (American Nurses' Association, 1983). Recently, she was honored by the Association of Rheumatology Health Professionals (a division of the American College of Rheumatology) with a Lifetime Achievement Award. She has been a part of Columbia Arthritis Center, Milwaukee, Wisconsin, since its inception in 1969. She now serves as nurse consultant to Smith-Pigg Consultants, Inc. She recently retired from her position as director of program development and outcomes studies for the Columbia Musculoskeletal Institute of Columbia Hospital.

Joe Selby is the assistant director for health services research in the Division of Research, Kaiser Permanente, Northern California. Selby is a family practitioner who cofounded and served as medical director of a federally funded neighborhood health center in Oakland, California, from 1976 through 1983. He has conducted epidemiologic studies of the etiology of non-insulin-dependent diabetes and its complications, as well as of insulin resistance and heart disease. He has also performed case-control studies of cancer-screening tests. Selby's health services section is responsible for evaluating and monitoring outcomes of care in the areas of mental health and substance abuse, asthma, neonatal care, breast cancer, and ischemic heart disease.

Victor Villagra is vice president of Medical Care Management at CIGNA Health-Care. His responsibilities include the strategic planning and implementation of care management programs. While at the Geisinger Health Plan, Villagra practiced internal medicine. In 1990, he received the Geisinger Clinician Investigator Award. In 1993, he created the Continuous Health Improvement Program of the Geisinger Health Plan and was named the program's medical director. He led the implementation of a variety of preventive and disease management programs across a large rural practice network.

Michael Von Korff is the associate director for research at the Center for Health Studies, Group Health Cooperative of Puget Sound. His major research interests are the management and outcome of depression and of chronic pain (back pain, headache, temporomandibular pain) among primary care patients. He is currently organizing intervention research on approaches to improving the self-management skills of patients with recurrent or chronic back pain. He has been working with the director of the Center for Health Studies on developing and evaluating generalizable models for managing chronic illness in staff-model HMOs.

Source: Institute for Research and Education.

address clinical process, organizational structure, and team member job performance."

Focus on the Patient

A good chronic disease management program must focus on the patient, above all. The clinician must inquire into the patient's expectations, experience, and perceptions. The more comfortable a relationship the clinician and patient have, the easier it will be for them to communicate about this key information. One issue that the doctor or nurse must communicate is that clinicians do not have all the answers or all the power. They cannot issue a diagnosis with absolute certainty or cure a chronic illness as they would "fix" an acute condition. These "deficits" could cause the patient to lose confidence in the health provider or treatment plan. If the clinician can help the patient understand these uncertainties, however, the patient can become motivated to study his or her own condition and, thus, to use this knowledge to compensate for the clinician's limitations. Making the patient central to treatment should be a goal for program design and implementation.

HALSTED HOLMAN: The patient is central to the management of chronic disease. You start off trying to find out what the disease means to them. How would they like it managed? What do they expect from you? From the visits? How can you fit their educational experience into their lives? It is really patient oriented. Physicians my age were all brought up to handle all patients stereotypically. What is your main complaint? When did it begin? And so forth. You were graded upon whether you did this list of things that essentially never asked the patient's opinion or any of the implications of the disease or its treatment to the patient.

KAREN MEYER: I think the number one thing that has to be there is a comfort level between the patient and me. If we have that comfort level, the patient will open up about many things. Central to the philosophy of our program is that the patient is the core of the team. Our philosophy is, "How can we help you? What are your goals?" If the patient tells me he or she only exercised two minutes a day—great, so be it. We may want ten minutes a day or more, but this is the patient's perception, and we keep building on that and nudging that ahead as the weeks go on.

HALSTEAD HOLMAN: It is important to raise the issue of uncertainty immediately, to explain to patients that there is a level of medical knowledge that does not allow anyone to give them absolute certainty about diagnosis. If they can come to grips with that notion (and my experience is that almost everybody can), they are much better off. They then say, "Well, what do I do about it?" And I say, "Learn to monitor yourself. Learn to pick up your trends. Here's the way to do it. If you need some help, we will provide that. But you become the observer so you can predict as well as I can where you're going and allow for your management to be precise." It is surprising, but they are able to deal with that.

It is a matter of introducing them to a different mind-set than they have. If they came in with a broken leg or a hot appendix, they would say, "Fix me," and you would say "I can. You should do this and this and this, and you're fixed." A different mind-set is required in the treatment of chronic illness.

JANICE SMITH PIGG: Particularly in chronic diseases where the diagnosis may not be certain early on, the patient must be helped to become comfortable with this uncertainty so as not to lose confidence in the health provider and treatment. In the inflammatory rheumatic diseases, exactly which one we are dealing with may not be obvious until the pattern of symptomatology and other criteria are evident over a period of time that not only can be months but may even be longer. But patients—as well as we as providers—like neat labels. So when it becomes more clear which systemic rheumatic disease is the one, and it is different than the one we might have initially thought the patient had, this new label can be very unsettling, with doubts about lost treatment time or the wrong treatment. This inability to categorize conditions neatly is contrary to what we like to think health care is. Patients need support and reassurance that the changing of names does not mean opportunity has been lost or treatment inappropriate, as they are based on disease processes.

Set Reasonable Goals

Adapting to a chronic illness usually takes time. For that reason, a chronic illness management program must be flexible enough to address each patient's stage in the disease process and the patient goals associated with that stage. Doctors and nurses should base a treatment plan on realistic expectations of what the patient can accomplish, and they should accept that patients will not always follow instructions. The trick is to demonstrate this acceptance to patients by praising the efforts they have made while encouraging them to comply more with recommendations.

KATHLEEN LOANE: The quality of my teaching of patients has changed over the years, based on what I learned from patients. I take what works for one patient and use it with another. I try to be very aware of what's going on and sensitive to what's happening in their lives. I try to develop a feeling of partnership. I try not to set them up for failure. I don't expect them to be 100 percent successful all of the time. If I am teaching adolescents, I know they are not going to do what they should do every day. So, I teach them that if they're fine for five days and quit, then just start over again. I try to get them to "buy in" in small stages.

I want them to feel well. I try to convince them that if they give me time and we work together, I can make them feel better. We will work together. I can't do it alone; it's you, me, and your primary care doctor. Sometimes I will say, "Give me three months and see where we can go. If you can do what I'm asking you to do at least 50 percent of the time or more, we can start." I tell them, "I can't cure you, I'm not going to cure you. I have drugs that control your asthma." Getting them to believe I am going to be there to work with them is important. They can call me if they have questions or if they can't start taking their medicine or if they forget. It's a partnership, and I state that right up front.

DONNELL ETZWILER: When we started with glucose monitoring, we thought patients wouldn't mind stabbing themselves four times a day if they saw an improvement down the line. I think we have to be very careful as professionals that we don't set up unrealistic expectations for these patients. You have to be able to pardon them if the person is doing only one or two tests. You say, "It looks like you're doing pretty well. Do you think we could do a little better if we had more data?" The data are not for the doctor; they are for patients themselves.

MICHAEL VON KORFF: In audiotapes of back pain patients, it is amazing that back pain patients bring up many things that they are doing, most of which are sensible. But it is very unusual for a physician to say, "That's great! You're doing exactly the right thing." This may be a more natural response for a nurse. The idea of starting from where the patient is, being satisfied with small steps, and recognizing change takes a while to occur, and there are going to be setbacks, is consistent with approaches that many nurse-educators take with patients. But these concepts are not part of the physician's life experience.

Focus Program Resources Where They Do the Most Good

In the interest of conserving limited resources, it is possible to classify patients by the severity of their illnesses and then to apportion care with a triage mind-set; sicker patients would fall under the category of case management, whereas others would receive less attention. This approach is problematic, however. Classifying patients requires certain information that clinicians simply may not have; for this reason, any classification may seem faulty. Patients' motivation levels should probably be taken into account. Why apportion resources to someone who will waste them? Or should that be the concern and responsibility of clinicians? Doctors and nurses can only make recommendations; they cannot force patients to comply.

VICTOR VILLAGRA: Patients who utilize a lot of resources generally are sicker. One model would simply look like a curve where a few severe cases would be triaged to predominantly case management. For those people, we do what we have talked about here. You know their names, it is a personal relationship, and you manage their care.

Others in the middle range of severity are not necessarily very sick or high utilizers of resources. They fall out of the domain of case management and enter the domain of programs (for example, community programs, work-site programs). These patients would include the mild asthmatic or the diet-controlled diabetic who is doing reasonably well. Patients in this cluster need some education. They end up getting their care from primary care providers, nurses, and so forth.

JOE SELBY: I suspect that the approach may differ from disease to disease. For diabetes, most of what a new model of care is supposed to do is secondary and tertiary prevention, and a lot of that is way down the road. You can't tell from what happened to the patient last year or even a year or two in a predictive model who's going to have the heart attacks and strokes ten years down the road. Yet you know that there are certain things that are going to have an impact on that. When you are doing a lot of secondary and tertiary prevention, it is tougher to focus in.

MARY PAT PAQUETTE: I think that one of the things you have to remember with case management is that nurses tend not to focus on one thing. If I have an asthmatic patient who also has a skeletal problem and needs something that day that has to do with orthopedics, I'm not just going to say, "Call your orthopod." I may actually get on the phone and talk with the orthopod. So case management tends to look at the broader picture, and I think that may address some of those issues. If a patient is considered high risk because there are extra issues or because his or her diabetes is out of control, case managers will attend to all of those things.

VICTOR VILLAGRA: I would concur with that. It is exactly what happens with some of the case managers I have worked with. The other issue is information. I frankly don't have information yet that tells me who are those two thousand who are not in my program—diabetics or asthmatics or whoever. I really have very little clinical information. But an administrative database can tell us who is utilizing a lot of resources. The classification into case management programs is usually a very fluid one. Some of the people who are in the case management strata are there just by being statistical outliers. I have not found tools to allocate patients through effective triage.

DONNELL ETZWILER: The concept of assigning or triaging patients gets us back to chronic disease and who's delivering the health care. The question is, Should patients identify what they want to do? For instance, in diabetes, if they want only maintenance therapy and are willing to risk the associated complications, that might be one program, and intensive therapy might be another. I have no problem if the patient has a 10.5 hemoglobin A_{1C}, and after I explain the complications, the patient tells me that she or he doesn't want to take care of her or his diabetes. If we have informed the patient of the associated risks, it is crazy for me to repeatedly pound my head against the wall the whole time when the patient just refuses to do it.

HALSTEAD HOLMAN: That's certainly my view. Patients should be offered opportunities, and those who appear by virtue of severity to be the most likely to benefit might be offered them more persuasively. But I certainly wouldn't go beyond that. In the last analysis, we are not responsible for the people who refuse to do those things that contemporary knowledge indicates are good and useful things to do. If they do them and they don't work for them and then they give up, that's fine with me. I don't quarrel with that, and I think we should continue to keep covering them. If they make no effort, then I don't see that we remain responsible. But I'm uneasy with that.

Combine Referral Guidelines with Clinician Judgment

Although there should be formal rules about when a primary care physician refers to a specialist, these rules should be followed with some give-and-take. The clinician making the referral should consider what the patient needs and who can best provide that. For instance, a nurse might be the best case manager for a common disease. A primary care physician might prefer to treat a complicated case at times. A specialist might be most appropriate for treating a rare disease. With each choice, there are some trade-offs and benefits.

JOE SELBY: Has anybody ever seen a formal guideline for when to refer? There was a flurry of interest in that not too long ago, and I have always had my doubts that you could formalize the referral decision, given the variation of skills of primary providers.

VICTOR VILLAGRA: We built that into a project, in part to pacify the specialists. We discussed the criteria for referrals to specialists with a primary care physician and allergist. They looked at them and said the rules were reasonable and agreed generally to follow those rules. Now, it was pointed out that the primary care physicians don't all have the same level of interest or competency in asthma. Some may prefer the flexibility to take treatment to levels that would "break" those rules (that is, treat more complicated cases themselves). I don't know if this is happening, but we're going to evaluate it.

Use a Team Approach

Effective chronic illness management requires a coordinated team approach (partnership) in the overall management of the patient's condition. The team members will typically include the patient, the family, physicians, nurses, and representatives from service organizations. A team approach makes treatment more comprehensive, because team members each contribute certain skills.

JOE SELBY: We think that we can gain a lot by replacing overburdened primary care physicians with interested nurse practitioners or diabetes nurse-educators who know how to manage the disease and who have a diabetologist to back them up. For a disease this common, the specialty modeling wouldn't work for the eighty-five thousand diabetics in the group. For a much rarer disease, that might be precisely the way to go.

I call it low-cost specialization when you replace the subspecialist with a nurse case manager who knows almost as much about that one basic disease. Patients get increased attention from somebody who knows more than the primary care physician and has easier access to telephone management and disease-specific information.

It is a lot easier to believe that this approach is going to work better than a primary care practitioner who has that same help from an information system (even support from an added member of the team). We would still be asking the primary care physician to take on not only diabetes but asthma and arthritis and back pain in this new intensive way in order to improve outcomes.

MARY PAT PAQUETTE: We have actually seen physician practice changes because of my influence. I see patients and families, and I assess and educate them. This takes some of the education burden off the physicians and provides another assessment of the family dynamics. I then consult with the primary physician. We discuss treatment, recommend changes as needed, and work on a plan of action we feel the family can handle. I think the physicians feel more comfortable giving more control to the families because of the increased education and follow-up. This is a team approach.

KATHLEEN LOANE: I think that the nursing role fits wonderfully. Pediatricians see a lot of patients within time limits, and chronic symptoms are not always picked up. An example is a child with exercise-induced asthma. This is a fine point that doesn't always come up in a routine examine, because family members aren't aware that they should bring it up or the clinician does not ask questions about it. But during the phone conversations or by monitoring patients, we can identify this and monitor by follow-up calls. If the symptoms are persistent and well documented, then the nurse can bring it to the attention of the physician, and things change. A great strength of nursing case management is that I was able to watch these patients over time and bring changes in the patient's condition to the attention of the doctor who then can make a decision.

Build Relationships with Patients

A chronic illness management model should encourage all team members to build relationships and develop trust. Consistent follow-up and communication with patients are critical to this effort.

MARY PAT PAQUETTE: Nurses need some back-up support for chronic disease management. As nurses, we listen a lot. We also do a lot of health promotion. Kathleen [Loane] and I both frequently teach patients not only how to take care of their disease but how to take care of themselves in general. We connect with the primary care physician frequently. The patient may meet with me once a week and with the primary care physician once a month. We try to bring them back to the primary care physician for health promotion. It's very important to keep the physician in the loop.

DONNELL ETZWILER: Chronic disease management really does not involve a lot of treatment; it is really maintenance. I think chronic disease treatment is closer to a nurturing concept, which physicians are not taught in medical school, at least when I was a student. If you do a procedure, you can make money. As pediatricians, we don't have a procedure, and therefore we get reimbursed for periods of time. It's not like popping out a cataract in half an hour and being reimbursed $1,000. You see patients with chronic diseases for years. The patient is not as appreciative of that attention, because it doesn't result in a sudden cure. I think that chronic disease patients really need nurturing.

KATHLEEN LOANE: We hired four nurses four years ago. When we did that, we looked for certain qualities that we thought were needed. Certainly, experience was desirable. What had they done in their careers in nursing? We didn't take people who had just staff experience but we looked for nurses who had done other things within their nursing careers showing autonomy. We looked for a commitment to be flexible. In our program, nurses carry beepers to respond quickly to clinicians and patients. It takes nursing to another level.

HALSTEAD HOLMAN: I see a modest number of patients who come to me referred by other rheumatologists with a referral letter, so they are looking for a second opinion. I would guess at least 50 percent of the time, if I say to the patient, "Now I have a letter from Dr. Jones, and I know why he sent you. Would you tell me why you came and what you want?" the response has nothing to do with what was in the referral letter. So there is really a substantial amount of miscommunication. The doctor is talking about doctor things, and the patient is talking about something else that has been missing in the prior relationship.

Give Patients Incentives to Modify Behavior

Patients need incentives to lead healthier lives. Education does not seem a sufficient motivator, and financial incentives are not ideal. Instead, patients need praise, at the very least.

VICTOR VILLAGRA: Empirically, I have observed that knowledge isn't enough. Not only is knowledge not enough but demonstrating that something works isn't enough. I know if I exercised regularly and if I lost five pounds, I would feel better. If the evidence is so convincing that this works, this ought to induce behavioral change. But this is not the case.

Once upon a time, the insurance companies paid for services and didn't ask anything. Then the liability was transferred to primary care physicians in the form of capitation. Thus, the insurance companies passed the risk.

Let's consider putting some of the financial responsibility on the patient—in a positive way. I don't know if it will work. I have looked at, for example, an array of incentive programs that have been put into effect in the workplace to promote lifestyle changes, and so forth. Some of them work very nicely, but some of them have been rather draconian and have had disappointing results in the long run.

DONNELL ETZWILER: We can change patient behavior by offering positive incentives or rewards, and it doesn't have to be money. It can be recognition. I think we can recognize patients in various ways. If nothing else, we can praise them for what they have done. We can change behavior by using identifiable rewards that are not necessarily monetary.

HALSTEAD HOLMAN: I would argue against using financial incentives. It would distract the attention of the providers away from the kind of information development and behavior change that they need to promote in order to do their job. I think it works in smoking because we don't know what else to do. I think we ought to have our feet put to the fire as health professionals in terms of changing to accommodate chronic disease.

Address Financial Issues, Along with Clinical Ones

When designing innovative programs, clinicians need to ensure that the ideas will not only improve care but also save money. The savings might be in the long term; an intervention might cost some money up front but prevent expensive hospitalizations. Money is not the only issue on clinicians' minds; they want to improve the process of care, patient satisfaction, and the medical outcome. They must, however, convince managed care organizations that their plans will save money overall.

VICTOR VILLAGRA: When we put together the asthma project, one of the critical questions in the planning stage was, What is so innovative and so clever about this that is worth testing and worth putting energy into? We discarded a few ideas because they were just not that innovative. There was, conceptually, nothing new. If we prove that a new initiative results in better care (improved health outcomes and reduced costs), then we have every intention of going to our commercial (fee-for-service) payers and saying that they really ought to pay for, for example, asthma medications, up front. It is going to cost them money, but the documented net effect of an intervention is positive. This assumes that patients play according to the rules that we set up. They have to go through the educational programs and demonstrate knowledge and skills in asthma self-care.

JOE SELBY: Well, let me ask you a question. Is there any program that you really could argue would be accepted if it doesn't either save money while holding outcomes the same, or improve outcomes in a moderate period of time, or improve process measures of care? Do people think that there are other reasons to implement a program, aside from those three reasons?

MICHAEL VON KORFF: Several of us have talked about system approaches that require fundamental changes in the way services are being delivered. In the short run, these changes may not save money or slow dramatic improvements in outcomes, but they may alter the long-term capacity of the system to manage chronic illness. If you have a system that has to reorient itself (for example, an information system), the payoff level may be modest in the short run, with considerable development costs, but in the long run it may create a capacity to support further change.

JANICE SMITH PIGG: We have taken initial steps to work with a managed care organization. There is suspicion on both sides, but more so of us and what we are trying to do. They were relying on claims data, and we were saying: "Let us show you things that you can implement that will improve quality and outcomes, as well as acceptance of your managed care program, because of increased patient satisfaction."

Implications for Improving Chronic Illness Management

The principles for successful chronic illness management models proposed by the expert panel are consistent with many of the points raised in the clinical and the management literature, or summarized in previous chapters. The panel members emphasized the need for involving patients in self-management and giving them motivation, the importance of drawing on a broad range of clinical expertise in supporting the patient, and the importance of coordinating and communicating through formal methods (such as guidelines for clinicians) and informal methods (such as building relationships with patients). They also underscored the necessity of designing cost-effective programs to win organizational and payer support.

The panel highlighted areas that have received less attention in previous chapters. Specifically, they noted that successful patient involvement and coordination of team activities depended, to a significant extent, on the interpersonal skills of the nurse-coordinator. They also raised issues about providing financial incentives to patients.

A Model Approach to
Chronic Illness Management

Now that we have looked at issues in designing and operating chronic illness management models and have studied the experiences of ongoing programs, we will condense these findings into the form of a "prototype" model. We do not regard this model as "ideal" in a clinical sense; that is, it is not necessarily the approach that a health care organization would adopt if resources were unconstrained. The model we propose, however, reflects the principles of chronic disease management described in Chapter Seven. At the same time, it has a reasonable chance of becoming an integral part of the real-world practice of medicine in which there are competing demands on clinician time and on organizations' financial resources.

In the first part of this chapter, we will discuss the assumptions that form the basis for the model. Then we will briefly describe each of the model's components as they relate to each other. After that, we will discuss the roles and responsibilities of the different members of the chronic illness team. With a patient "flow chart," we will explore further how the model would function from the health care organization's point of view. Finally, we will identify critical issues relating to model design.

Underlying Assumptions

Several important assumptions underpin our model. In most respects, these assumptions closely parallel the principles for designing and operating a chronic illness management program.

- Given the multiplicity of resources and individuals involved in treating chronic illness, some variation of a health care team approach is necessary for effective patient care.

- Communication and coordination within the health care team are critical for success. This suggests that some team member should assume a coordinator or liaison role.

- The workloads of primary care physicians are high and will continue to grow. A chronic illness management model will need to be structured so as not to add to those workloads.

- The patient must do much of the work of chronic illness management. Therefore, the model must create support for the patient in this role. It will not be sustainable unless patients feel supported.

- Clinicians' abilities to be effective managers in the context of a chronic illness management model will vary. Therefore, programs should teach clinicians how to function as leaders on chronic illness management teams.

- In an era of constrained resources and managed care, it is critical to measure and report performance. This is the only way to ensure the long-term survival of chronic illness work groups. The organization will need to devote ongoing resources to evaluations of model effectiveness.

These assumptions have guided our model development. In some ways, they constrained model design; we rejected model components that were not consistent with these assumptions. In other respects, they identified areas that required special attention. In effect, they forced decisions with respect to model design and emphasis that we might otherwise have avoided.

Essential Components

As shown symbolically in Figure 8.1, the patient is the model's focal point. The patient provides care and has desires that guide the team's efforts to manage the illness. To a great extent, the team's success will be measured by the patient's satisfaction. Therefore, the chronic illness management model is consciously patient centered.

Figure 8.1. Chronic Illness Management Model.

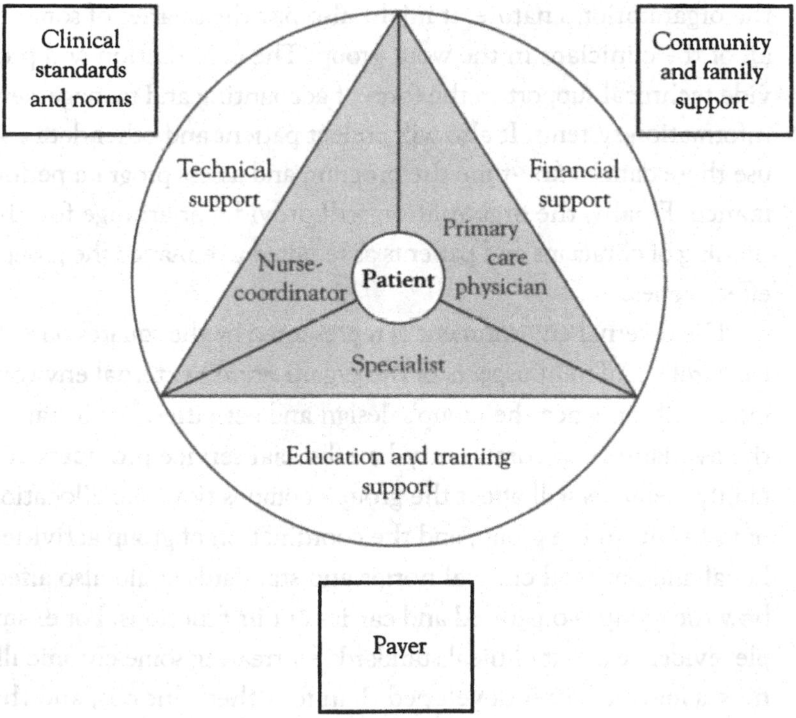

Source: Institute for Research and Education.

The triangle and the surrounding circle represent different organizational levels. The triangle contains the patient, along with team members who are employed by, or affiliated with, the principal medical care organization. These individuals include the nurse-coordinator, the primary care physician, and any specialists with expertise in the chronic illness. In some cases, the triangle may encapsulate the entire chronic illness management team. In other cases, however, the team may include social services providers and family members, depending on the patient's needs and the availability of these resources.

The circle around the triangle represents the larger organization that supports the team's activities. The team needs three types of support from this larger organization: financial, technical, and educational. The organization will provide the physical space and subsidize the initial costs of program implementation. Depending on the organization's nature, it might also pay the salaries of some or all of the clinicians in the work group. The organization will provide technical support in the form of accounting and management information systems. It also will collect patient and other data and use these data to fine-tune the program and assess program performance. Finally, the organization will provide, or arrange for, the training of clinicians and patients as required to enhance the group's effectiveness.

The external environment is represented by the squares outside the circle. Different aspects of the organization's external environment will influence the group's design and activities. For instance, the availability of community-based social service providers and family members will affect the group's composition, the allocation of tasks within the group, and the coordination of group activities. Local and national clinical norms and standards could also affect how the group is organized and carries out its functions. For example, evidence about clinical standards for treating some chronic illnesses may be better developed than for other illnesses, and this could influence the degree to which work groups rely on formal (for example, guidelines) versus informal (for example, conversations) methods of communication and coordination. Finally, the external environment ultimately provides the financial resources to carry out the work group's activities. If those who purchase health care believe in the group's value, they will be willing to reimburse health care organizations or clinicians for the time and resources devoted to work group activities. Each of these environmental features can change over time through interactions between the organization and the environment. For instance, purchaser attitudes may be influenced by evidence about work group effectiveness, and family members' willingness to participate in the group may increase through educational efforts.

Team Members' Functions and Roles

It is important to define clearly the necessary skills, functions, and operational roles of each group member. The most important team member, the patient, must want to learn about the disease and be willing to participate in its management. The patient also needs to be able to communicate effectively with other team members about the impact of the chronic illness on his or her daily life. For the primary care physician, specialist, and nurse-coordinator, effective and empathic listening and communication skills are essential when working with patients, family members, and other team members. Clinicians also need a desire to work as part of a team in managing the patient's care, a working knowledge of guidelines applicable to treating the chronic condition, and experience and skill in educating patients, families, and other staff. Table 8.1 lists various functions that a chronic illness team will need to perform. It also identifies the team members who might be involved in each function.

Patient Identification

According to Table 8.1, the first task in forming a chronic illness management group is deciding that the patient is a good candidate.

Table 8.1. Team Members' Functions.

Operational Functions	Patient	Primary Care Physician	Specialist	Nurse-Coordinator	Family	Organization	Community Agencies
Patient Identification							
• Identifies patients for program (via utilization review, diagnosis code, guidelines, patient or family request)	X	X	X	X	X	X	
Diagnosis and Assessment							
• Initial assessment of medical status and intensive medical management		X	X	X			
• Obtains functional status assessment, lifestyle assessment, psychosocial assessment, caregiver assessment	X			X	X		
• Gains understanding of patient's goals in managing chronic illness	X	X	X	X	X	X	
Treatment and Monitoring							
• Directs treatment and monitoring decisions based on patient's medical status and needs		X	X	X			
• Refers or self-refers to specialist for diagnosis, intensive medical treatment, and follow-up as needed	X	X	X	X	X		
• Assesses status of patient referred (by primary care physician or self-referred) and begins intensive treatment		X	X				
• When patient is stabilized, refers patient back to primary care physician (or nurse-coordinator) for further education, ongoing follow-up, and monitoring			X				
• Refers to program for follow-up and monitoring		X	X				
• Periodically assesses and reevaluates patient's functional status, medical status, psychosocial status, and goals		X	X	X		X	X

	C1	C2	C3	C4	C5
Maintains contact with nurse-coordinator regarding patient condition	X	X	X		X
Schedules ongoing follow-up and monitoring of patients according to treatment plan	X	X	X		X
Is available for case reviews with other clinicians via phone calls or scheduled meetings	X	X	X		
Coordinates and participates in case reviews		X	X		
Meets with primary care physician, specialist, patient, and family to review assessment findings and develop a treatment plan		X	X		
According to "nurse guidelines" (developed by specialist and primary care physician), refers patient to primary care physician or specialist for new or ongoing, unresolved problems	X	X	X	X	
Interacts with other nurse-coordinators, office nurses, and physicians about patient's concerns when appropriate		X	X		
Follows through with treatment plan (takes medications, attends appointments, and so on)	X				
Supports and encourages patient	X	X	X	X	X
Follows treatment plan for caring for patient		X	X	X	X

Communication

	C1	C2	C3	C4	C5
Documents findings and medical treatment plan for providers, patient, and family	X	X	X		X
Documents follow-up in medical chart	X	X	X		X
Communicates with providers regarding condition and its impact on patient functioning (social, physical, mental)	X		X	X	X
Communicates with providers regarding patient's		X	X	X	X

Table 8.1. Team Members' Functions, continued.

Operational Functions	Patient	Primary Care Physician	Specialist	Nurse-Coordinator	Family	Organization	Community Agencies
condition and family members' ability and willingness to provide support and assistance	X						
• Communicates to providers the barriers to complying with treatment (medicine's side effects, conflicts in schedule for treatment activities, and so on)				X	X		X
• Asks questions of providers to gain understanding of chronic condition and impact on patient's lifestyle	X			X	X		X
• Communicates the treatment and follow-up strategy to patient and family		X	X	X			X
Education: Patient and Family							
• Provides education to patient and family members on the chronic condition and its impact on patient's and family's lives		X	X	X		X	X
Education: Provider							
• Attends professional education sessions		X	X	X		X	
• Serves as educational resource for staff			X				
• Provides expertise in developing treatment guidelines for primary care physicians and nurse-coordinators		X	X				
• Meets regularly with other nurse-coordinators to share experiences and case studies				X			

• Attends educational sessions or seeks educational experiences regarding specific chronic illness (focusing on two to three chronic conditions)			X
Organizational Support			
• Long-term commitment of organizational resources to chronic disease management	X	X	
• Willingness to modify existing organizational structures (for example; clinic staffing, phone system, information system) to support chronic illness management efforts		X	
• Support data collection on patient status and outcomes to be used in feedback to provider and patients		X	X
Program Evaluation			
• Periodic assessment and reevaluation of functional status, psychosocial status, medical status, patient goals	X	X	
• Provides information on costs of care			X

Source: Institute for Research and Education.

How do clinicians identify patients who will benefit from participating in such a group? Depending on the scope of the group's activities, the group can find and select patients with the following resources:

1. Data from the organization's information system (including diagnostic codes; records on the utilization of services, such as hospitalization, clinic visits, and pharmacy purchases; and patient demographics) that indicate which patients qualify for treatment

2. Criteria established in care providers' guidelines or work group guidelines that indicate which patients are appropriate

3. Referrals by primary care physicians, specialists, or nurse-coordinators after diagnosis and assessment of appropriateness

4. Requests for treatment by the patient or family

Diagnosis and Assessment

To diagnose and assess the patient, the primary care physician or specialist must evaluate the patient's medical status, with the nurse-coordinator's assistance. In addition, the nurse-coordinator may work with the patient and family to assess the patient's functional status, lifestyle, and psychosocial status, as well as any caregiver issues. The initial assessment gives the patient the opportunity to define goals for managing the illness over time, which is valuable information for team members. Clinicians and the organization will also gain baseline information to use in assessing the care's effectiveness over time. With the results of the initial assessment and evaluation, the patient and care providers then develop a plan to meet the patient's specific needs.

Treatment and Monitoring

The primary care physician directs the ongoing medical management based on the patient's medical status, goals, and needs. The specialist collaborates in this effort in the following ways:

• By clarifying issues pertaining to complex diagnoses

- By providing intensive therapy in order to stabilize patients before they enter the care model or as they need it thereafter

- By providing periodic consults and case reviews with the nurse-coordinator or primary care physician as the patient's status changes

- By educating patients, primary care physicians, and nurse-coordinators about ongoing developments in the treatment of the illness

A plan for treating the patient and continuing to monitor progress is developed with input from the nurse-coordinator, patient, primary care physician, and specialist. The plan addresses the goals that the patient has specified for managing the illness's impact on his or her life over time. It is critical that all team members have a clear understanding of the patient's goals throughout the treatment and monitoring process.

The nurse-coordinator has primary responsibility for ongoing follow-up and monitoring based on the care plan. In this respect, the nurse will provide educational opportunities for the patient and family members on issues relating to the chronic condition and to self-management skills; support and encourage the patient; perform periodic assessments of the patient's functional, psychosocial, and medical status; and review patient goals to ensure that the patient's needs are being met. In order for the care model to be effective, patients must be motivated and willing to participate in implementing the care plan. The nurse-coordinator may need to enlist family members' or caregivers' help in encouraging the patient. Community agencies, such as home care services, may also need to participate in the plan's implementation.

Communication

It is important for patients to tell health care providers about any barriers to their compliance with the treatment plan. Patients also need to be willing to ask questions about their condition and to identify their goals for managing the chronic illness, including the desired level of functioning they wish to achieve or maintain.

The physicians and the nurse-coordinator are responsible for documenting the initial assessment results, the treatment strategy, and the information collected from follow-up visits or phone contacts. The nurse-coordinator has a key role in ensuring that communication is complete and current among clinicians, patients, family members, and other outside agencies. This is critical to maintaining, evaluating, and adjusting treatment plans in response to patients' changing needs.

Education

To provide patients with education means supplying information about the chronic condition and its impact on the patient's lifestyle, as well as training in self-management skills. Physicians and nurse-coordinators can provide education during clinic visits through one-on-one sessions with the patient; conferences with the patient, family, and other care providers; and group education and support sessions facilitated by the nurse-coordinator. The health care organization, or divisions within the organization, can support this effort by offering seminars for patients and family members on topics related to specific conditions. Education strategies for patients with chronic illnesses need to be continuous and flexible in order to address patients' changing needs as they experience the illness's impact on their lives.

All the care providers should make an effort to attend professional conferences or internal organizational education sessions. Through these methods, they can increase their knowledge of current methods of treating and managing the chronic illness. The health care organization needs to show strong support for professional education.

Organizational Support

An important foundation for developing and implementing a model of chronic illness management is the organization's long-term commitment and willingness to support new models of care. Organizations should be willing and able to modify existing structures, such as phone systems and information systems; handle staffing issues related to new team members' roles and responsibilities; revamp reimbursement mechanisms; and support any data collection or retrieval to be used in program evaluation or feedback to providers and patients.

Program Evaluation

There are two levels of program evaluation. First, data must be collected for the ongoing assessment of the patient's medical, functional, and psychosocial status, as well as a review of patient goals in light of the patient's current health status. These regular evaluations involve the patient, the nurse-coordinator, physicians, and family members. The results of these periodic assessments may trigger the need for short-term, intensive treatment by the specialist; a change in the care plan; or additional patient education concerning the chronic illness, its treatment, and the patient's self-management. An evaluation may also identify the need for outside services, such as home care.

The second level of evaluation addresses how well the model of care has worked in a particular health care system. Overall program evaluation includes measuring the impact of the care model on patients, assessing patient and provider satisfaction with the care model, and determining the program's cost-effectiveness. This evaluation will be used in determining whether this model of chronic illness management improves the patient's care and in documenting its cost.

Process of Care

The flow diagram in Figure 8.2 depicts how a patient interacts with the health care organization under the chronic illness management model. For example, suppose a woman is newly diagnosed with

Figure 8.2. Patient Flow Diagram.

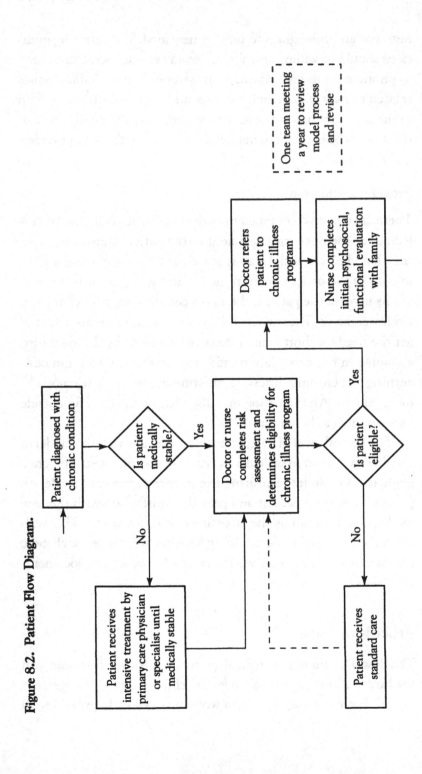

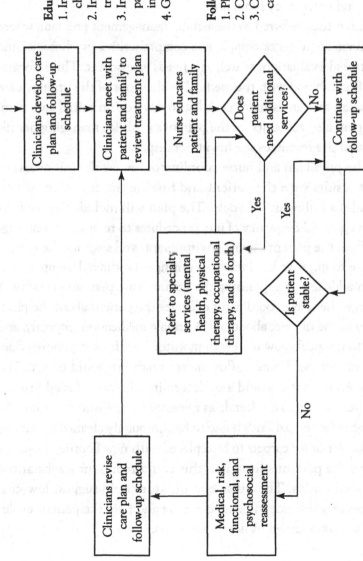

Education includes
1. Information about chronic condition
2. Information about treatment
3. Information about patient and family roles in self-management
4. Goal setting

Follow-up includes
1. Phone calls by nurse
2. Clinic visits to see nurse
3. Clinic visits to see primary care physician or specialist

Clinicians develop care plan and follow-up schedule

Clinicians meet with patient and family to review treatment plan

Nurse educates patient and family

Does patient need additional services?

Yes

No

Continue with follow-up schedule

Refer to specialty services (mental health, physical therapy, occupational therapy, and so forth)

Is patient stable?

Yes

No

Medical, risk, functional, and psychosocial reassessment

Clinicians revise care plan and follow-up schedule

Source: Institute for Research and Education.

asthma. After the diagnosis is established and the patient is determined to be medically stable, the physician and nurse-coordinator jointly determine her eligibility for participation in the program. They base this decision on established criteria that indicate which patients will benefit from this model of care management. These criteria include the asthma patient's medical history and past inpatient and emergency room use.

She is then referred to the asthma management program, where the nurse-coordinator completes a comprehensive psychosocial and functional evaluation, as well as a needs assessment. This information is combined with the medical evaluations of the primary care physician and an asthma specialist to develop an initial care plan. The plan also accounts for the patient's goals for managing her illness and the resources she has at her disposal.

The physician and nurse-coordinator review the initial assessment results with the patient and finalize the care plan, which includes a follow-up schedule. The plan will include the medication's type and frequency of use, procedures to remove asthma triggers from the patient's living environment, and steps for the patient to take to improve her breathing during an asthma flare-up.

In addition to explaining the asthma care plan and treatment strategy, the nurse-coordinator educates the patient about the physiology of the disease, about how to inhale medications properly, and how to use peak-flow meters to monitor breathing capability. Specific objectives for peak-flow meter readings would be set. The nurse-coordinator would also determine the need for additional resources and make referrals as necessary. For instance, it may be desirable for the patient's house to be thoroughly cleaned to remove pet dander or for carpets to be replaced with new flooring. Depending on the patient's situation, this could represent a substantial financial outlay. The nurse-coordinator could suggest low-cost sources of assistance in house cleaning and help the patient evaluate the cost of different flooring options.

After this initial visit with the patient, which could last as long as two hours, the follow-up phase begins. During this phase, the nurse-coordinator regularly communicates with the patient by telephone to monitor her progress and answer her questions. During these conversations, the nurse-coordinator might collect data on peak-flow meter readings, reinforce proper procedures for administering inhaled medications, check on the frequency and timing of the patient's breathing problems, and encourage changes in the patient's living environment. Patient visits to the primary care physician or specialist could also be scheduled as needed.

If at any time the patient's condition unexpectedly changes, or if new issues relating to the treatment plan arise, the nurse-coordinator can contact the primary care physician or specialist and initiate a reassessment. This reassessment may suggest a need for intensive therapy for a short period of time, possibly with a stronger medication, or a change in care plan and monitoring schedule (for example, more frequent peak-flow readings).

The emphasis is on flexibly meeting patients' requirements. As they suffer from a chronic disease, they may experience periods during which they have acute care needs. Despite these times of heightened requirements, patients should need little intensive medical intervention if the chronic illness management program provides effective support. For an asthma patient, this means avoiding hospitalizations, emergency room visits, and medications with potentially adverse side effects whenever possible.

Critical Issues in Model Design

We believe that the model we have presented can be used successfully in a variety of health care settings. Some issues relating to components of the model design are likely to arise in many health care organizations, however.

Facilitating Communication Among Team Members

Communication among work group members is vital for coordinating care delivery, alerting clinicians about changes in patient condition, educating clinicians and patients, and gathering information for assessing work group performance. Although communication can be organized and carried out in many different ways, both formally and informally, we believe health care organizations must structure communications so that they impose a minimal burden on physicians. Only in that way can the model become an integral part of primary care physician practice. In many care management models, all the care team members (excluding the patient) meet regularly to review the patient's status and progress. This type of approach is not likely to be feasible for primary care physicians in most practices. If primary care physicians view communication demands as excessive, they will resist model implementation and the proposed model will not be sustainable over time. Instead, communication with primary care physicians must be carried out on a more informal, as-needed basis.

Aspects of the model support this objective. First, the nurse-coordinator can facilitate communications among team members, freeing the primary care physician from this role (Evans, 1994). Second, placing a nurse in the coordinator role, and giving the nurse training supplemented by treatment guidelines where appropriate, means that the coordinator will be able to exercise independent judgment on many care-related questions. This reduces the time required of the primary care physician. Third, decentralizing the model by placing (or selecting) the nurse-coordinator in the primary care physician's office enhances opportunities for informal communications that do not disrupt the primary care physician's normal practice schedule.

A second communication issue relates to the need to support, educate, and listen to the patient on an ongoing basis. For a patient-centered model to work, the patient must function as an integral part of the care process. To facilitate this, patients should communicate with clinicians as needed, rather than waiting for regularly scheduled appointments or acute flare-ups of the chronic illness. This type of communication is most likely to happen if a supportive, trusting relationship exists between the patient and the nurse-coordinator. One way to build such a relationship is for the nurse to call the patient. During the phone call, the nurse can offer support; solicit information about medication compliance and other critical treatment issues; and identify physical, social, or financial barriers to treatment (Roberts and others, 1995).

An issue that arises in this context is determining the appropriate number of patients that can be linked with any single nurse-coordinator. If a nurse-coordinator cares for too many patients, it may not be possible for them to develop the strong relationship that leads to effective communication and patient participation in the care process. We believe nurse-coordinators should have other responsibilities in the primary care practice, in addition to their roles in chronic illness management work groups. This enhances the model's integration into the primary care practice and limits the number of patients that any given coordinator can serve.

We recognize, however, that two risks are associated with this strategy. First, the nurse-coordinator may experience divided loyalties associated with playing different roles in the practice. Having other demands can limit the time the nurse can devote to chronic illness management. Second, nurse-coordinators can come under pressure from the health care organization to increase their case-loads with the objective of enhancing the model's apparent cost-effectiveness. Although measured cost-effectiveness might improve in the short run, as the nursing coordinator's salary is distributed across more patients, effectiveness may deteriorate in the longer term; work groups may function less effectively because of inadequate patient-coordinator communication.

Dealing with Patient "Ownership" Issues

For chronic illness management work groups to function effectively, they must confront and overcome any "patient ownership" issues that arise for primary care physicians or specialists. In their practices, primary care physicians assemble panels of patients and arrange for the care of these patients. From the standpoint of many primary care physicians, the role of other clinicians is to provide support and expertise that help them manage "their" patients. In treating patients with severe chronic illnesses, specialists sometimes function in this same way by providing "principal care" (see Chapter Two). In theory, they assume responsibility for a panel of patients and arrange for, or coordinate, care from other providers as needed.

Either of these situations could lead to feelings of patient "ownership"—that is, a reasonably clear distinction between "my patient" and "your patient." This view is reinforced by the way in which physicians are compensated. In a fee-for-service payment arrangement, physicians are paid for each unit of service they deliver. This creates incentives to retain, rather than "share," patients, because collaborative treatment approaches can result in reduced income. Even in multispecialty group practices, in which physicians are primarily salaried, there may be financial incentives that work at cross-purposes to the adoption of team care approaches. For instance, salaried physicians may be required to see a targeted number of patients in a given period, and they may receive bonuses for encounters in excess of target levels.

In effect, both by acculturation and reimbursement, physicians are discouraged from adopting collaborative, team approaches to care delivery in real-world practice settings. One way for organizations to try breaking down the "my patient, your patient" mind-set in implementing chronic illness management work groups is through clinician education concerning work groups' objectives and functioning. By defining physician roles clearly, emphasizing the potential for improving patient care and satisfaction, and demonstrating high-level administrative support for the model, organizations may be able to create the "our patient" mentality that is critical for successful model implementation.

These activities by themselves are not likely to be sufficient, however. Reimbursement arrangements must also be restructured so that primary care physicians are not penalized financially for participating in chronic illness work groups in which care that physicians once delivered is provided by nurse-coordinators or by patients themselves. The exact nature of this restructuring will vary across health care organizations, but it is likely to depend partly on the degree to which payers can be convinced that redesigned reimbursement arrangements will not increase their overall expenditures for care.

Financing Implementation and Ongoing Operations

Implementing a chronic illness management model requires an initial investment on the part of the health care organization. This investment is likely to be greatest for organizations that are early adoptors of the model and substantially less for "followers." Funds will be needed to do the following: develop educational materials for clinicians and patients; design and test assessment instruments; modify management information systems capabilities or install separate information systems to support nurse-coordinators; identify patients who might potentially benefit from the model; and subsidize the salaries of nurse-coordinators and other clinicians whose contributions to care may not be fully reimbursable initially. Organizations that are followers may be able to reduce their initial investment costs by using, with minor modifications, the educational materials, assessment instruments, and information systems that early adopters develop.

More critical to the model's sustainability over time is the health care organization's ability to cover ongoing operating costs. The way in which the organization views this problem will depend, to a considerable extent, on the way in which it receives payment for care.

If most of its revenues come from capitated payments, the operating costs associated with the model will need to be built into the capitated rate. Alternatively, the model will need to be justified based on its ability to deliver care of comparable quality with similar levels of patient satisfaction but at a lower cost than usual care. If the model increases costs, the additional benefits that it generates for patients will need to be emphasized, in the hope that payers will be willing to cover these costs through higher capitation rates. In either case, the organization has a strong incentive to be very careful in documenting and analyzing costs and outcomes continually.

In contrast, if the organization receives most of its revenues on a fee-for-service basis, funding the model is likely to be viewed as a problem of maximizing overall reimbursement for the services provided. In this case, a critical issue will be which services are grouped together for reimbursement purposes. In particular, the organization's ability to secure fee-for-services reimbursement for the various activities of the nurse-coordinator will be critical. This may depend on whether payers view the nurse-coordinator's services as being provided under the physician's direct supervision or independently of the doctor.

Irrespective of how these issues are resqlved, the organization must be prepared to demonstrate that the model delivers comparable care at a lower cost to payers, or that it improves patient outcomes and satisfaction sufficiently to justify any additional costs that the payer incurs (Zalta, Eichner, and Henry, 1994). As is the case under capitation payment, organizational resources will need to be devoted to tracking and analyzing the expenditures and outcomes associated with care delivery.

Educating Clinicians and Patients

Virtually all chronic illness management models emphasize educating patients about disease symptoms and phases, as well as self-management techniques (for example, Greenfield, Kaplan, and

Ware, 1985). Clinicians teach patients informally in one-on-one meetings and in more formal group sessions for patients and family members. Both clinicians and patients recognize the need for both initial and ongoing patient education. Supportive patient educational materials are widely available for most chronic illnesses, and health care organizations can acquire them at minimal cost. Resources may need to be devoted, however, to training clinicians in the use of these materials and the use and appropriateness of different teaching techniques. Typically, nurse-coordinators will not resist this training, and patients are normally receptive to learning more about their chronic illnesses, particularly right after the diagnosis.

In contrast, a second element of education is not addressed systematically in chronic illness management models. That element may be harder to implement in health care organizations. It involves teaching clinicians to be better managers and coordinators of patient care. As we have seen, chronic illnesses are often medically complex and involve multiple individuals in their treatment, with a central role for patients. This places somewhat different care management demands on clinicians than they encounter in treating acute illnesses. It is essential for group members to communicate and coordinate their activities for treatment to be cost effective. Maintaining work group members' active participation and commitment over an extended period can also be a critical issue. In general, the work group must be effectively managed for the patient to benefit to the maximum extent possible from any chronic illness management model.

Although certain management skills are intuitive for some people, in general it is not realistic to assume that clinicians who are competent by virtue of their clinical training will also be competent managers. Training clinicians in such areas as group process, communications, and the management of work flows would likely improve the day-to-day functioning of chronic illness management work groups.

Large health care organizations may already provide periodic educational opportunities about these and related topics for select employees. For other organizations, this may represent a new area of human resource development. Organizational management will need to be convinced that this sort of education is important, because it will require an ongoing investment of organizational resources. It also may be necessary to sell clinicians on the importance of this training for improving patient care, because it will be a departure from more familiar types of continuing education.

Evaluating the Model's Success

Assessing the performance of chronic illness work groups will pose several challenges for health care organizations. As noted previously, a group's impact on patient functioning and health status may be difficult to detect (especially in the short run), the "perfect" comparison group is unlikely to exist, and the evaluation effort itself will be costly. We assume, however, that a credible, reasonably complete evaluation of model performance will be necessary, at least initially, so that the health care organization and purchasers will accept the model. Some form of ongoing performance review will also be critical for identifying areas of the program to improve.

With respect to the initial evaluation effort, it will be important to include both short-term and intermediate measures of program implementation and its effects on patients so that the burden of assessing program effectiveness does not rest entirely on clinical and health status outcomes. Table 8.2 lists possible areas to address in program assessments. Of particular importance for most health care organizations will be the measurement of patient satisfaction. If patients are not pleased with the model, it is unlikely that clinicians will accept it, even if it reduces costs compared with "usual care." Patient satisfaction is an outcome that the model is likely to influence in the short run. It is an important marker for decision makers in the health care organization and for purchasers. If a "patient-centered" model for chronic illness management does not improve patient satisfaction in the short run, it is unlikely that patients will accept it in the long run, even if patient clinical outcomes demonstrably improve.

A second area of satisfaction that needs to be addressed in an evaluation relates to clinician satisfaction with the model. Although the model's impact on patients is the ultimate concern, that impact is less likely to be positive if clinicians do not value the model. Clinician satisfaction could serve as one short-term measure that is likely to be correlated with long-term model acceptance by the health care organization.

The multiple assessment areas listed in Table 8.2 represent different types of model impacts, each important in its own right. One way to assess the model's performance is to track different measures

Table 8.2. Areas to Address in Program Assessment.

Process Measures
- Degree to which model has been implemented
- Proportion of eligible patients receiving service under the model

Clinician Satisfaction
- Care patients receive
- Roles, responsibilities, and relationships

Patient Satisfaction
- Access to care
- Quality of care
- Role in managing illness
- Organizational support
- Interactions with clinicians
- Family's role
- Health status
- Overall care

Patient Functioning
- Physical
- Social
- Mental

Costs
- Direct medical care
- Indirect patient and family
- Program-related

Source: Institute for Research and Education.

in each of these areas over time after the model is implemented. This would provide a general picture of how patients are doing, as well as an estimate of what it is costing the organization, and patients, to implement the model. If costs are minimal (or fully reimbursable), or if impacts on patients are obviously beneficial and substantial, this simple tracking exercise may provide sufficient information to decision makers within the health care organization.

It is not clear that this always will be the case, however. It seems more likely that decision makers will want to know what would have happened in the absence of the model. That is, did the model increase or reduce costs? Did it improve or decrease patient satisfaction relative to usual care? Answering these types of questions requires that the evaluation include a credible comparison group whose members receive "usual care," defined as the care patients would have received without the model.

Health care organizations have three options for establishing such a comparison group. In some ways, the simplest option is to conduct a before-and-after analysis, in which the group of patients with a specific chronic illness serves as its own comparison group. Data are collected for these patients for a period of time before the model is implemented and then for a similar length of time after implementation. Using this approach, patients' "before" experiences represent treatment without the model.

There are at least two possible drawbacks to this approach, one methodological and one practical. First, from a methodological standpoint, it may not be appropriate to equate a "before model" experience and a "without model" experience. The preimplementation care patients received could differ from the care they would later have received without the model. The longer the pre- or postimplementation periods used in the assessment, the more likely it is that this would be the case. Second, to assess the impact of a chronic disease management model, a relatively long evaluation period may be more desirable. From a practical standpoint, however, collecting data may not be desirable before implementation because it could interfere with successful model implementation. Once a health care organization commits to a new approach to chronic illness management, it may need to build on the momentum generated by this commitment and move directly into model implementation. If so, this could preclude the collection of "before" data through patient surveys. The before-and-after evaluation would then be limited to data available retrospectively through administrative records or medical charts.

Another option is to create a "contemporaneous" comparison group through a controlled phase-in of the model at different care sites, assuming that the health care organization offers primary care at multiple, geographically distinct locations. In this case, the experience of chronically ill patients at the comparison sites (those primary care practice sites without access to the model) could be contrasted with the experience of similar patients at the model sites. The underlying assumption would be that the comparison site experience was a reasonable approximation of the model site experience in the model's absence.

Again, there are potential methodological and practical drawbacks to this approach. Methodologically, there may be any number of reasons that the experience at the comparison sites would not represent the experience at the model sites had there been no model. For instance, the process of care delivery could differ systematically across the two groups of sites in ways that could affect patient experience, irrespective of the model's effect on patients. Observed differences in patient experiences would be attributed to the model but would actually reflect these preexisting site differences. From a practical standpoint, a structured phase-in may not be administratively possible. It might be politically difficult for a health care organization to "sell" the model's potential advantages to one group of clinicians and patients while withholding the model from other clinicians and patients.

A third option is to construct a comparison group from patients served by a different health care organization. Obviously, the same types of methodological considerations arise. From a practical standpoint, this approach is likely to be extremely difficult and time consuming to implement unless there is already a high level of trust and a history of cooperation between the two organizations.

Some of the methodological problems of relying on before-and-after comparisons or contemporaneous comparisons can be addressed by combining these approaches. That is, before-and-after data would be collected in the comparison sites and in the model sites. Unfortunately, this approach is likely to be even more difficult for most health care organizations to implement.

The discussion to this point has addressed ways to define measures and design an evaluation plan. A related matter is, Who should collect the data and carry out the evaluation? The answer depends in part on the audience for the evaluation results. If decision makers internal to the organization are to use the results (perhaps to decide whether or not to continue or expand the model or to make decisions about fine-tuning it), then the health care organization itself can collect and evaluate the data. If, however, the primary audience for the evaluation consists of decision makers external to the organization (for example, purchasers), they might doubt the credibility of a self-evaluation. In this case, the health care organization may want a collaborative arrangement with external evaluators; the organization's employees could help the evaluators collect data and interpret results.

The drawback of this approach is that the organization loses some control over the evaluation. The evaluators may interpret the data or present the results in ways that the health care organization feels are inappropriate. Each health care organization implementing a chronic illness management model will need to judge whether the potential advantages of collaboration with external evaluators—presumably greater objectivity and credibility—are sufficient to outweigh the loss of control and the additional costs incurred.

Implications for Improving
Chronic Illness Management

The chronic illness management model we propose includes a prominent role for a nurse-coordinator; emphasizes patient education and self-management; recognizes the social, as well as medical, dimensions of the illness; and suggests some variant of a team care approach. The team would have defined roles for primary care physicians, specialists, nurse-coordinators, social service providers, and family members who would support and collaborate with patients. These features of the model are intuitively appealing and consistent with expert opinion about desirable principles for care delivery.

Some features of the model do raise fundamental organizational and professional issues concerning the practice of medicine, however. These issues include the possible need to redefine the roles of primary care physicians versus specialists and of nurses versus physicians in the treatment of patients. Similarly, the model might mean redefining patients' responsibilities relating to their own care. It could also mean restructuring compensation schemes to reward clinicians appropriately for "shared work." Addressing any one of these issues could create a substantial impediment to the model's implementation within a health care organization.

Health care organizations should address potential implementation problems in two ways. First, the program design should include organizational, as well as clinical, considerations relating to chronic illness management. Second, organizations should plan the implementation process carefully. In the concluding chapter, we discuss how health care organizations can assess their organization's readiness to implement a chronic illness management model similar to the one proposed in this chapter.

9

Considering Whether an
Organization Is Ready to Change

This chapter (and the subsequent Appendix) should help organizations assess how ready they are to restructure chronic illness care processes. We believe that such an assessment is a critical component in any effort to rethink chronic illness management within a health care organization. The organizational assessment approach we propose can also be employed to monitor progress in changing care processes and to identify areas that need ongoing management attention.

Our approach to assessing organizational readiness is based on our experience in implementing a pilot hypertension management model. We believe that the best way to examine operational issues, and to devise strategies for addressing them, is through a sequential implementation process. During this process, technical issues relating to model operations can be identified and different solutions attempted.

This approach has its limitations, however, as it will not identify problems that can arise only when broad-scale implementation is attempted. For instance, patient monitoring and data collection within the organization may require a different approach under broad-scale implementation than when the model is implemented at a small number of sites. Also, if there is internal opposition to adopting the new model, it may not become evident until implementation is organizationwide. Finally, a staged implementation process may dissipate initial organizational enthusiasm and support for the model and reduce its overall impact on the organization if implementation drags on over a long period.

Although very little has been written specifically about operational issues relating to the restructuring of medical care processes, numerous organizational management books have addressed the redesign of business processes to increase effectiveness. This literature offers a variety of different conceptual lenses, any of which could be used in assessing organizational readiness. As a framework for our assessment approach, we have adopted (with some modifications) the three-level approach of Rummler and Brache (1995). These authors argue that organizations must be managed at the level of the organization, the work process, and the individual job or performer. In this chapter, we pose questions about organizational readiness at each of these levels.

In the Appendix, for each of the questions posed in this chapter, we add a series of subquestions. By answering the specific subquestions, decision makers can assess whether their particular organizations are ready to restructure treatment processes for chronic illnesses. They can identify where it is possible to make changes that would enhance organizational readiness. The Appendix also summarizes the responses to the subquestions in the form of an organizational scorecard. This scorecard provides an overview of how the decision maker perceives organizational readiness at all three levels. The scorecard can help in developing an organizational implementation strategy.

Organization Level

The *organization level* refers to relationships between the organization and the external world, including relationships with entities that provide revenue to the organization. It also includes relationships among the major functional areas within the organization. For a health care organization, external issues include relationships with those who purchase services, whereas internal issues include management of relationships among broad functional areas (such as care delivery, finance, MIS, and so forth). The organization's overall goals are set at the organization level, along with strategies to accomplish these goals and resource allocation decisions to support the implementation of these strategies. Several critical questions relating to organizational readiness need to be addressed at the organization level.

1. *Is the effective management of care for chronically ill patients an important part of the organization's overall mission?*

The organization is more likely to support restructuring the care process for chronically ill people if serving this population is a central part of the organization's mission. In contrast, if serving those with chronic illnesses is a small part of the overall mission, it will be more difficult to sustain organizational commitment and obtain the organizational resources necessary to restructure care processes.

2. *Does the restructured care delivery program have sufficient time to meet organizational goals and prove its effectiveness?*

The treatment of most chronic illnesses is expected to be ongoing and will not necessarily result in a cure. The objective is to alter the illness's course, thereby improving the patient's quality of life. Care process restructuring may require a significant initial investment, with benefits (in either improved patient health or cost savings) accruing gradually. If the organization can only risk trying out a new program for a short time, there may be little chance of garnering organizational support for changes, given this configuration of benefits and costs.

The amount of time an organization allows for programs to show payoffs is likely to depend on its financial condition and its competitive position in the market. Organizations that are struggling financially may be open to restructuring care processes and thus may seem receptive to new approaches for chronic illness treatment.

These organizations, however, may value only those innovations that promise a quick fix for their financial problems. For this reason, they may not be able to sustain, over the longer term, the restructuring of chronic illness treatment.

3. *Do the goals of functional areas within the organization, and the strategies being used to achieve those goals, support the restructuring of chronic illness treatment processes?*

Functional areas within the organization have their own performance goals and certain strategies for attaining those goals. Goals and strategies within each functional area should be examined for their ability to accommodate the demands that restructuring care processes will impose on the system.

As an example, the information systems functional area within an organization may have an explicit short-term goal of upgrading the organization's billing process (for example, submitting all bills within five days of service delivery) and may have allocated all possible internal resources to achieve this goal. In this case, there may be no resources available to develop information capabilities to support new treatment processes. Alternatively, if the goal of the information systems functional area is to support the improvement of clinical care processes in the organization, this could indicate an organizational readiness to develop information systems that would help nurse-coordinators and physicians communicate better, thus supporting team approaches to chronic illness treatment.

4. *Are purchasers willing to pay for restructured care processes for chronic illness? Is reimbursement for restructured care processes possible under existing payment procedures?*

Improvements in chronic illness care processes may result in increased costs to the organization, at least in the short run. To secure reimbursement of these costs, it will at least be necessary to demonstrate improvements in patient health and satisfaction with care. Even so, purchasers may not be willing to pay more for better outcomes.

If the organization receives most of its revenues through capitated payments, it will either have to pass on any additional costs to payers in the form of higher rates or justify them to payers based on projected future cost reductions. To the degree that market pressures constrain capitated rates, changes in care processes that reduce short-term costs are likely to receive the strongest organizational support. On the other hand, if the organization receives most of its revenues on a fee-for-service basis, a critical issue relates to the ability of the organization to secure fee-for-service reimbursement for the various activities of the nurse-coordinator. This may depend on whether payers view nurse-coordinators as working under a physician's direct supervision or as acting independently of the physician.

5. *Is the organizational culture supportive of coordinated, team approaches to patient care?*

In many health care organizations, the issue of who "owns" patients can assume major importance for primary care physicians and specialists. Chapter Eight noted that in organizations with deeply embedded clinical structures or with compensation arrangements that support a "my patient, your patient" view of the care process, it will be difficult to restructure chronic illness care processes using collaborative treatment approaches. Such approaches are more likely to be successful in organizations that can create an "our patient" mentality through a supportive mission statement and a clear articulation of goals and that take strong management actions to resolve "turf" issues.

Many multispecialty group practices are strongly oriented toward having specialists manage chronic illnesses. The primary care physician's role is defined, explicitly or implicitly, as primarily that of a referral agent. Under these circumstances, major emphasis may be placed on medical aspects of treating chronic illnesses, and there may be little perceived need for a team approach to care. Within any organization, the specialist's usual role can vary for different chronic illnesses and may depend on the historical development of the group practice as much as on the characteristics of different chronic illnesses.

Assessments of organizational culture will need to examine subgroups within the organization, as well as the organization as a whole. For instance, in one group, asthma specialists may see a major collaborative role for primary care physicians in treating that illness, whereas cardiologists may not see a similar role for primary care physicians in treating stable coronary angina. In another group, this culture might be reversed. In most groups, however, one would expect that primary care physicians would play a dominant role in treating hypertension in all but the most severe cases of this disease.

Process Level

The *process level* refers to the level of the organization at which the critical work is accomplished. Within a health care organization, the "process" at issue is delivering care to patients or to defined populations of enrollees. Redefining the process of caring for the chronically ill means reconfiguring the resources devoted to their treatment. Organizational readiness for restructuring chronic care processes must be assessed at the process level, as well as the organization level.

1. *Can the existing process of caring for the chronically ill be clearly described? Can its shortcomings be identified? Is the need for restructuring clear, in light of these shortcomings?*

Changes in care processes can require substantial adjustments at every level within the organization. Individuals in the organization—whether managers, clinicians, or patients—are unlikely to support these changes in the long term unless a clear need for change can be demonstrated in measurable terms. For example, say that it can be convincingly documented that an organization's usual hypertension treatment process succeeds in controlling blood pressure a relatively low percentage of the time. Clinicians in that organization are likely to support efforts to restructure care. This would not be as true for clinicians in organizations that have no documentation on the effectiveness of care. Support for restructuring hypertension treatment is also more likely if someone identifies the particular shortcomings of existing care processes and shows how a restructured process can improve care. In practice, this may not be an easy task, because usual care can vary across sites within an organization, resulting in a lack of agreement about the shortcomings of usual care.

2. *Can agreement on reasonable performance targets for the restructured care process be reached, in light of the perceived shortcomings of the existing process?*

In order to design and implement an effective restructuring of care processes, it is necessary to be able to specify in measurable terms what the restructuring will accomplish. These goals may be stated at a process level (for example, the number of hypertensive patients who are served in a given time period) or at a population level (for example, the proportion of hypertensive patients in a care system who have their blood pressure under control).

Even if a consensus on the shortcomings of usual care can be reached, there may be disagreement within the organization about reasonable goals for a restructured care process. Those charged with implementing the restructuring effort may argue for flexible goals that can be easily modified along the way. For instance, proponents of restructuring may argue for the goal of increasing the number of visits by patients with uncontrolled hypertension. Goals of this nature can be useful in measuring the degree to which the care process is altered, but they provide little information about the degree to which patients value the new process and ultimately experience improvements in well-being, relative to usual care.

3. *Can key individuals within the organization who will be affected by a restructured chronic illness treatment process be recruited to participate in that restructuring?*

In order to restructure the care process, a work group or steering team should be formed to carry out implementation activities. The steering team should include key individuals within the organization who must give their support or resources so that restructuring can take place. Management should hold the steering team accountable for achieving the goals established for a restructured care process.

4. *Is there a "process owner" who will assume leadership responsibility in the restructuring process?*

Top management within the organization must play an active, ongoing role in order for significant process restructuring to occur. A "sponsor" or "owner" of the restructuring effort is needed to guide the steering team, remove organization-level obstacles to restructuring, and secure needed organizational resources and support at key times.

Identifying a potential process owner within an organization sounds simple but can be complicated in practice. In organizations that have well-defined management structures and stable leadership, the right process owner may be obvious. Even in these organizations, however, it may be unclear how high a rank a process owner should have within the organization's management structure. Furthermore, in many health care organizations, considerable instability in management structure and leadership results from acquisitions, mergers, and network relationships. Individuals who occupy key leadership positions, and who could be effective process owners, may not remain in these positions long enough to provide needed guidance and support. The need to replace a process owner could greatly prolong efforts to restructure chronic illness treatment processes.

5. *Do all relevant individuals within the organization appreciate the need to devote resources and time to a carefully staged implementation process? Are there likely to be sufficient time and resources available for implementation?*

Restructuring the delivery of chronic care within a health care organization inevitably challenges core beliefs and long-standing roles. Redesigning chronic care processes is an essential first step in accomplishing change, but actually implementing redesigned processes within the organization is likely to require the greater commitment of time, resources, and management attention. Organizations that do not appreciate this and that are not committed to supporting a significant and potentially extended implementation effort are less likely to restructure chronic care processes successfully.

Purchasers and policymakers are challenging health care organizations to rethink care processes and demonstrate value. In an effort to respond to these demands, administrators may feel compelled to implement new initiatives and programs at a rapid rate. Guidelines development, health promotion and prevention programs, and total quality improvement efforts are examples of health care organizations' initiatives in this regard.

If organizations are rewarded in a visible way for undertaking such efforts, they may devote their administrative efforts and resources to developing new responses to market demands. Unfortunately, this will mean that past initiatives are not implemented effectively. Rolling out new initiatives is glamorous and can generate accolades for the organization; implementing programs is messy and may receive little external reinforcement.

6. *Is there commitment to having patients meaningfully involved in their own treatment?*

People with chronic illnesses provide a substantial amount of their own care. Therefore, for restructured care processes to be successful, patients' support and involvement are critical. This support is most likely to be present when patients are part of the health care team and when they help design chronic illness treatment processes. The success of the restructured treatment process should be assessed, in part, by patient satisfaction. Ironically, organizations that most need to rethink chronic illness care processes may well be those that have paid the least attention to patient involvement in the past. In these organizations, clinicians are likely to be committed to a traditional model of care, with the patient as "care recipient." They may pay lip service to the importance of patient involvement but resist attempts to redefine the patient role in a meaningful way.

Job or Performance Level

The *job or performance level* refers to the people who deliver care for chronic illnesses and the tasks or jobs involved in delivering that care. It concerns the skills, training, and responsibilities of team members, including the patient. Restructuring care delivery for chronic illnesses inevitably changes the work environment of team members and others in the organization who are asked to support the team's activities. This restructuring also changes relationships between patients and clinicians and between different types of clinicians (for example, specialists and primary care physicians). It is important to assess the organization's readiness to support or facilitate changes at the job or performance level that are necessary for successfully restructuring chronic illness treatment.

1. *Assuming that a nurse-coordinator position is created as part of the restructured treatment process, can measurable goals for the nurse-coordinator be established? Do the organization's compensation policies allow nurse-coordinators to be compensated for achieving goals?*

The nurse-coordinator is a key individual in the chronic illness management team, but most health care organizations will have little experience with this position. Because the position is not familiar within the organization, goals and expectations for nurse-coordinators will need to be clearly articulated. Nurse-coordinators will have stronger incentives to work toward these goals if their compensation depends, at least in part, on the degree to which they achieve goals.

2. *Are there constraints on the organization's ability to select individuals with appropriate skills and training to fill nurse-coordinator positions?*

Effectively, nurse-coordinators must possess a variety of interpersonal skills to complement their clinical expertise. Nurse-coordinators need to facilitate communications among team members, develop strong linkages to patients, and be able to educate patients effectively about their roles in the redefined care process. The nurses already employed at primary care practice sites may not possess all the skills they need to be effective nurse-coordinators; it may be necessary to recruit individuals from outside of the practice for these positions. Different health care organizations may face constraints, however, in recruiting appropriate individuals for nurse-coordinator positions. For instance, organizations that are reducing staff in some areas may want to shift nurses whose jobs have been eliminated to newly created nurse-coordinator positions. If considerations such as these become dominant in the recruiting process, the individuals hired may not have the skills that nurse-coordinators need.

3. *Will the organization commit the resources to training and education that the restructured care process needs to function effectively?*

Both clinicians and patients widely recognize the need for initial and ongoing education of chronically ill patients. Resources may also need to be devoted to training clinicians to be better managers and coordinators. This may represent a new area of human resource development, and organization managers may need to be convinced of the need to invest resources in it.

4. *Do existing compensation systems discourage clinicians from participating in chronic illness treatment teams? Can systems be designed and implemented to reward clinicians and patients for team participation?*

Physicians must refer patients to nurse-coordinators and have an ongoing collaboration about treatment for a team approach to be viable. In determining compensation levels, health care organizations must be willing to give physicians credit for participating in overall treatment processes, even when the physician does not directly provide units of service. Ideally, nurse-coordinators should receive compensation for providing care to a designated panel of patients and for helping patients achieve measurable goals rather than for seeing a high number of patients in a given time frame. At least initially, patients can be encouraged to manage their own illnesses through modest, direct financial incentives (for example, reduced copayments). In the longer term, the team's support of the patient may be sufficient to ensure patient participation in the care process.

5. *Should individuals within the organization who are not directly part of the care team have their incentives and responsibilities changed in order for the restructured care process to be effective? Can these changes be implemented?*

Because the delivery of care is the central function of any health care organization, attempts to restructure care processes inevitably affect individuals with an indirect connection to treatment processes. These individuals may resist the restructuring of chronic care processes if it adds to their workload without any commensurate change in rewards. This resistance can be a critical impediment to restructuring if it comes from individuals whose skills are essential to the new care delivery approach or if it occurs at critical junctures in the implementation process.

There are many possible ways in which restructuring chronic illness treatment processes could affect jobs in a health care organization. For example, nurse-coordinators need to communicate with specialists and primary care physicians about their interactions with patients. To facilitate this communication, the nurse-coordinator can dictate visit notes. The dictated notes will be transcribed and put in the patient's medical record. If the transcription department's budget is being reduced, however, or if the department is trying to meet existing transcription demands with fewer resources, staff members are likely to resist the new chronic illness treatment approach; it will increase their workloads with no change in compensation or unit budget. Whether such resistance will impair the restructuring initiative depends on whether nurse-coordinators have alternative, reasonably priced methods of maintaining records and communicating with other clinicians (Christianson and others, 1997).

Implications for Improving Chronic Illness Management

In this chapter, we have posed and discussed a series of questions. They all relate to a health care organization's readiness to restructure its approach to chronic illness treatment. Because care delivery is the central "work" that health care organizations perform, any attempt to restructure care delivery processes will raise complex issues. It will affect virtually everyone in the organization to varying degrees. For this reason, designing a conceptually sound chronic illness treatment model is only a first step in improving care delivery. Attention and resources must also be devoted to implementing the model within the constraints imposed by the care system and its external environment.

Appendix

Assessing Organizational Readiness for Restructuring Chronic Illness Management

In Chapter Nine, we identified and discussed general issues about organizational readiness to restructure chronic care processes. In this Appendix, we revisit these issues in the context of an organizational assessment tool. For each of the questions posed in Chapter Nine, we present subquestions. By answering these questions, decision makers can assess how ready their organization is to restructure chronic illness treatment processes. They can identify possible barriers to change and begin to formulate strategies to use in overcoming these barriers.

Organizational Level

1. Is the effective management of care for chronically ill patients an important part of the organization's overall mission?

The mission is clear.

No

Yes

- In what way is the mission statement unclear?
- Can the mission statement be obtained? From whom?

Mark where the organization is on this scale:

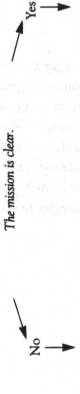

It's a primary focus of the organization's mission.

It's not an essential part of the organization's mission.

If the organization's rating is in the shaded half of the scale then answer the following questions:

- Is the organization's mission statement under review?
- Is the organization receptive to expanding the existing mission statement?
- Is there a reasonable likelihood that the revised mission statement will include care of patients with chronic illnesses?

2. Does the restructured care delivery program have sufficient time to meet organizational goals and prove its effectiveness?

The time frame for accomplishing goals is clear.

No

Yes

• Are goals and objectives unclear?

• Are goals and objectives clearly stated, but the time period for achieving them is unclear?

• Can the appropriate time horizon for judging program success be clarified? Who could provide this clarification?

Mark where the organization is on this scale:

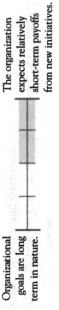

Organizational goals are long term in nature.

The organization expects relatively short-term payoffs from new initiatives.

If the organization's rating is in the shaded half of the scale then answer the following questions:

• Are exceptions ever made to this general expectation?

• How likely is it that a restructured chronic illness care process would be viewed as an exception?

3. Do the goals of functional areas within the organization, and the strategies being used to achieve those goals, support the restructuring of chronic illness treatment processes?

The goals of functional areas are clear.

No →

Yes →

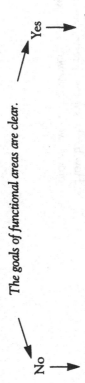

- For which functional areas are goals not stated clearly? Are strategies unclear?
- Can a clearer statement of goals or descriptions of strategies be obtained?

Mark where the organization is on this scale:

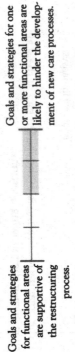

Goals and strategies for functional areas are supportive of the restructuring process.

Goals and strategies for one or more functional areas are likely to hinder the development of new care processes.

If the organization's rating is in the shaded half of the scale then answer the following questions:

- How important are these functional areas to the successful implementation of restructuring? Is there a lack of clarity concerning how goals or strategies of specific functional areas might affect restructuring? Is it possible to acquire the information needed to reduce ambiguity?

- Are goals and strategies in these areas internally consistent? Could any inconsistencies be exploited to support restructuring?

- Are goals and strategies under review? Is there a way to provide input to the revision of existing goals and strategies to make

4a. Are purchasers willing to pay for restructured care processes for chronic illness?

Purchaser attitudes are clear.

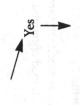

No

- What mechanisms are available to assess the attitudes of purchasers?

- Are there resources and is there an organizational commitment to carry out an assessment?

Yes

Mark where the organization is on this scale:

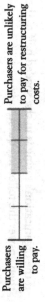

Purchasers are willing to pay.

Purchasers are unlikely to pay for restructuring costs.

If the organization's rating is in the shaded half of the scale then answer the following questions:

- What are purchasers' concerns? Can these concerns be alleviated in the design phase of restructuring?

- Is it likely that purchasers can be convinced of the value of restructured care processes?

- What points will be effective in convincing purchasers? How should arguments be presented?

4b. Is reimbursement for restructured care processes possible under existing payment procedures?

Existing payment procedures are clear.

No →

- Is the position of nurse-coordinator new in the organization, or are nurse-coordinators currently receiving reimbursement for the provision of services?
- What is the required supervisory role for the physician as it relates to reimbursing nurses for the provision of services?

↑ Yes →

Mark where the organization is on this scale:

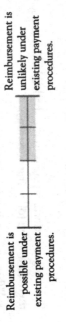

Reimbursement is possible under existing payment procedures.

Reimbursement is unlikely under existing payment procedures.

If the organization's rating is in the shaded half of the scale then answer the following questions:

- Is the reason for likely denial of reimbursement clear? Is there a process for changing reimbursement procedures? For appealing denial?
- Can features of a restructured care process be altered to increase the likelihood of reimbursement?

5. Is the organizational culture supportive of coordinated, team approaches to patient care?

The existing organizational culture is clear.

No →

Yes →

- Have similar efforts been attempted in the past? Are they relevant for assessing organizational culture?

- Are there subunits within the organization that are clearly supportive of team approaches? What is their influence within the organization? Are they likely to reflect the organization's overall culture?

Mark where the organization is on this scale:

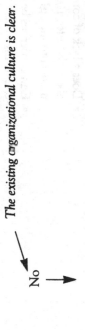

The culture is supportive.

The culture is not supportive.

If the organization's rating is in the shaded half of the scale then answer the following questions:

- How important is the culture in understanding the behavior of this organization?

- What specific elements of organizational culture are not supportive of team approaches?

- Are these elements changing or susceptible to change?

Process Level

1. Can the existing process of caring for the chronically ill be clearly described? Can its shortcomings be identified? Is the need for restructuring clear, in light of these shortcomings?

The existing care process is clear.

Yes →

Mark where the organization is on this scale:

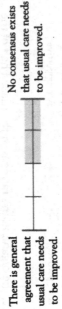

There is general agreement that usual care needs to be improved.

No consensus exists that usual care needs to be improved.

If the organization's rating is in the shaded half of the scale then answer the following questions:

- Does a lack of consensus reflect conflicting evidence about the effectiveness of usual care? Is some evidence more convincing?
- Can consensus be achieved through a closer examination of existing evidence and care processes? Or is there fundamental resistance to assessing existing chronic illness care processes?

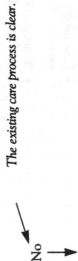

No →

- Does the lack of clarity about the process of usual care reflect a lack of information? Can information about usual care processes and their impact on patients be gathered at a reasonable cost?
- Are there multiple processes of usual care that result in different perceptions about performance? Can these perceptions be reconciled?

2. Can agreement on reasonable performance targets for the restructured care process be reached, in light of the perceived shortcomings of the existing process?

Targets can be specified in measurable terms.

No →

Yes →

- Is the inability to specify targets related to an inability to identify shortcomings in the existing process or an inability to quantify shortcomings in measurable terms?

- Would more information about the existing process assist in specifying targets in measurable terms?

- Is there uncertainty about whether targets should be patient-specific or population-based?

Mark where the organization is on this scale:

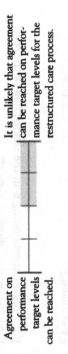

Agreement on performance target levels can be reached.

It is unlikely that agreement can be reached on performance target levels for the restructured care process.

If the organization's rating is in the shaded half of the scale then answer the following questions:

- Does a perceived inability to reach agreement on target levels signify more fundamental resistance to restructuring? Do conflicts within the organization about targets reflect fundamental differences with respect to organizational mission?

- Could a formal consensus-building process lead to agreement on target levels? Would the appropriate parties agree to participate in such a process?

3. Can key individuals within the organization who will be affected by a restructured chronic illness treatment process be recruited to participate in that restructuring?

Identification of key individuals is possible.

→ Yes

No →

• Is it impossible to identify these individuals because of a lack of understanding about the effects of a restructured care process?

• Can at least some key individuals be identified? Can initial restructuring proceed with these key individuals?

Mark where the organization is on this scale:

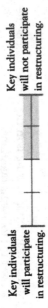

Key individuals will participate in restructuring.

Key individuals will not participate in restructuring.

If the organization's rating is in the shaded half of the scale then answer the following questions:

• How many and which key individuals are unwilling to participate?

• Does resistance to participation reflect employment insecurity, overcommitment in other activities, indifference, or other factors?

• Can resistance be overcome with management encouragement or educational efforts? What inducements to participation can be offered?

4. Is there a "process owner" who will assume leadership responsibility in the restructuring process?

Potential process owners can be identified.

No →

Yes →

- Is the process owner role unfamiliar for managers within the organization?
- Is there ambiguity about who would be an appropriate process owner? About who could identify appropriate process owners?

Mark where the organization is on this scale:

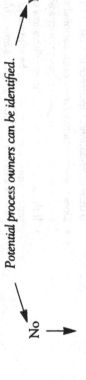

The appropriate process owner is likely to agree to a leadership role.

It is unlikely that the appropriate process owner can be convinced to assume leadership.

If the organization's rating is in the shaded half of the scale then answer the following questions:

- What are the obstacles to recruiting a process owner?
- Is there instability at the upper-management level of the organization? Other?
- What strategies can be pursued to overcome the obstacles identified above relating to the recruitment of a process owner?

5. Do all relevant individuals within the organization appreciate the need to devote resources and time to a carefully staged implementation process? Are there likely to be sufficient time and resources available for implementation?

There is a clearly recognized need to devote resources to implementation.

No

- Is the lack of clarity due to lack of knowledge about the implications of a restructured chronic care treatment process? Can clarification be obtained from organizational management?
- Is there disagreement within the organization about the goals and objectives of the new process? Can anything be done to resolve this disagreement?

Yes

Mark where the organization is on this scale:

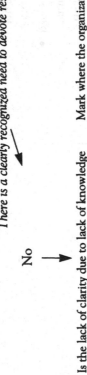

Adequate resources and time are available for implementation.

The resources and time available for implementation are unlikely to be adequate.

If the organization's rating is in the shaded half of the scale then answer the following questions:

- Does the insufficiency reflect a lack of information regarding the resources and time needed for implementation? What can be done to construct accurate estimates? Is there organizational experience that can inform this process?
- Does this insufficiency reflect organizational resource constraints that are unlikely to change, or a low organizational priority assigned to implementation?
- If the lack of time and resources reflects low organizational priority attached to restructuring, can management be convinced to reorder priorities? Will resources be allocated to restructuring if it assumes a higher priority in the organization?
- What are likely to be the most important constraints? Time of key actors? Limitations on other resources? Other?

6. Is there commitment to having patients meaningfully involved in their own treatment?

The proposed role of the patient in a restructured care program is understood.

No →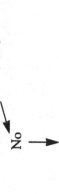

- What means are available to assess the level of understanding within the organization of the patient's proposed role in the care process?
- Can the patient's role in the restructured care process be explained more effectively? What issues inhibit understanding?

Yes →

Mark where the organization is on this scale:

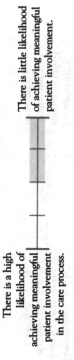

There is a high likelihood of achieving meaningful patient involvement in the care process.

There is little likelihood of achieving meaningful patient involvement.

If the organization's rating is in the shaded half of the scale then answer the following questions:

- Does this unlikelihood represent widespread organizational resistance to patient involvement? A lack of historical precedence? Both?
- Can organizational indifference or resistance to patient involvement be overcome through educational efforts and management support?
- How important is patient involvement in the initial implementation stages? Can commitment to patient involvement be expected to build over time within the organization?

187

Job or Performance Level

1. Assuming that a nurse-coordinator position is created as part of the restructured treatment process, can measurable goals for the nurse-coordinator be established? Do the organization's compensation policies allow nurse-coordinators to be compensated for achieving goals?

Measurable goals can be articulated.

Yes →

No →

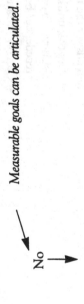

- Is there disagreement about the means by which nurse-coordinator performance should be measured? What is the nature of the disagreement? Is there a mechanism for resolving the disagreement?
- Is there disagreement about whether achievement of nurse-coordinator goals can be quantified? Can agreement be reached on appropriate *indicators* of goal achievement?

Mark where the organization is on this scale:

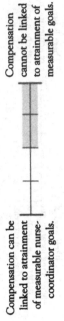

Compensation can be linked to attainment of measurable nurse-coordinator goals.

Compensation cannot be linked to attainment of measurable goals.

If the organization's rating is in the shaded half of the scale then answer the following questions:

- Are there organizational policies that inhibit the linking of compensation to measured achievement of quantifiable performance goals? How relevant are these policies for this effort? Can exceptions be made?
- Is resistance from potential nurse-coordinators likely to be a factor? Are there ways to structure compensation to minimize resistance while retaining a link to goal achievement?

2. Are there constraints on the organization's ability to select individuals with appropriate skills and training to fill nurse-coordinator positions?

It is clear which skills and training are needed.

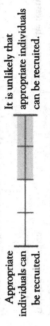

No

Yes

- What aspects are unclear? Is there experience within the organization with similar positions that would provide useful information about needed skills and training?

- Does the lack of clarity reflect an inadequate description of performance expectations? Of the nurse-coordinator role in a restructured treatment process?

Mark where the organization is on this scale:

Appropriate individuals can be recruited.

It is unlikely that appropriate individuals can be recruited.

If the organization's rating is in the shaded half of the scale then answer the following questions:

- Is there a shortage of individuals with appropriate skills and training in the community? Can individuals be attracted from outside the community?

- Are there constraints that require hiring individuals from within the organization? Can these restraints be removed? Is there a shortage of individuals with appropriate skills and training in the organization?

- Can training programs be developed that would impart the necessary skills to individuals who might be appropriate for the position?

3. Will the organization commit the resources to training and education that the restructured care process needs to function effectively?

The types of training and educational activities required are clear.

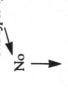

No

- Is the lack of clarity related to an inadequate understanding of roles and responsibilities? What can be done to enhance the understanding of roles and responsibilities?
- Is the lack of clarity related to a deficit of evidence that relates training activities to measurable skill enhancement? What types of evidence are needed? What are the likely sources of this evidence?

Yes

Mark where the organization is on this scale:

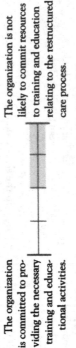

The organization is committed to providing the necessary training and educational activities.

The organization is not likely to commit resources to training and education relating to the restructured care process.

If the organization's rating is in the shaded half of the scale then answer the following questions:

- Is the organizational culture supportive of training and educational activities?
- Is the organization committed to training and educating patients but not clinicians? Or vice versa?
- Are appropriate training and educational activities available within the organization? What are the barriers to accessing them?

4. Do existing compensation systems discourage clinicians from participating in chronic illness treatment teams? Can systems be designed and implemented to reward clinicians and patients for team participation?

Existing compensation systems can be easily described and are understood by the clinician.

No →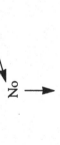

Yes →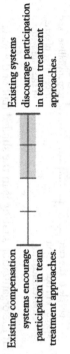

- What elements of existing compensation schemes are unclear? How can they be clarified?
- How are incentives in existing systems communicated to clinicians? Do special efforts need to be made to communicate these incentives?

Mark where the organization is on this scale:

Existing compensation systems encourage participation in team treatment approaches.

Existing systems discourage participation in team treatment approaches.

If the organization's rating is in the shaded half of the scale then answer the following questions:

- What elements of existing systems are the least amenable to change? Are these elements critical to the encouragement of participation?
- Is it possible to make incremental changes in existing systems?
- Who has the authority to change existing systems? Is that person supportive of restructuring chronic illness treatment processes?
- Will the process leader be supportive of changes in existing compensation systems?

5. Should individuals within the organization who are not directly part of the care team have their incentives and responsibilities changed in order for the restructured care process to be effective? Can these changes be implemented?

The responsibilities of other individuals are clear.

No →

Yes →

- What other individuals are likely to affect the success of the restructuring efforts?
- Can information be obtained regarding their job responsibilities and incentives, as they relate to a restructured care process?

Mark where the organization is on this scale:

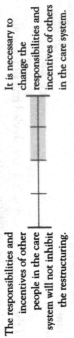

The responsibilities and incentives of other people in the care system will not inhibit the restructuring.

It is necessary to change the responsibilities and incentives of others in the care system.

If the organization's rating is in the shaded half of the scale then answer the following questions:

- What are the major barriers to implementing the needed changes? How can opposition to change be overcome?
- Is the organizational sponsor or some other appropriate individual willing to work for the necessary changes?
- If the problem pertains to a single individual or unit, can implementation be structured to minimize the participation needed from that individual or unit?

192

Organizational Scorecard

Decision makers can use the organizational scorecard to synthesize their responses to the questions on the previous pages. This scorecard provides an overview of organizational readiness to restructure chronic illness treatment processes, and it can help decision makers develop strategies to overcome barriers to change.

	Readiness of Organization 1 Yes 2 Uncertain 3 No	Importance as Barrier to Change 1 Not important 2 Somewhat important 3 Very important
Organization Level		
1. Is the effective management of care for chronically ill patients an important part of the organization's overall mission?		
2. Does the restructured care delivery program have sufficient time to meet organizational goals and prove its effectiveness?		
3. Do the goals of functional areas within the organization, and the strategies being used to achieve those goals, support the restructuring of chronic illness treatment processes?		
4a. Are purchasers willing to pay for restructured care processes for chronic illness?		

	Readiness of Organization 1 Yes 2 Uncertain 3 No	Importance as Barrier to Change 1 Not important 2 Somewhat important 3 Very important
4b. Is reimbursement for restructured care processes possible under existing payment procedures?		
5. Is the organizational culture supportive of coordinated, team approaches to patient care?		

Process Level

	Readiness of Organization	Importance as Barrier to Change
1. Can the existing process of caring for the chronically ill be clearly described? Can its shortcomings be identified? Is the need for restructuring clear, in light of these shortcomings?		
2. Can agreement on reasonable performance targets for the restructured care process be reached, in light of the perceived shortcomings of the existing process?		
3. Can key individuals within the organization who will be affected by a restructured chronic illness treatment process be recruited to participate in that restructuring?		
4. Is there a "process owner" who will assume leadership responsibility in the restructuring process?		

5. Do all relevant individuals within the organization appreciate the need to devote resources and time to a carefully staged implementation process? Are there likely to be sufficient time and resources available for implementation?

6. Is there commitment to having patients meaningfully involved in their own treatment?

Job or Performance Level

1. Assuming that a nurse-coordinator position is created as part of the restructured treatment process, can measurable goals for the nurse-coordinator be established? Do the organization's compensation policies allow nurse-coordinators to be compensated for achieving goals?

2. Are there constraints on the organization's ability to select individuals with appropriate skills and training to fill nurse-coordinator positions?

3. Will the organization commit the resources to training and education that the restructured care process needs to function effectively?

4. Do existing compensation systems discourage clinicians from participating in chronic illness treatment teams? Can systems be designed and implemented to reward clinicians and patients for team participation?

Readiness of Organization	Importance as Barrier to Change
1 Yes 2 Uncertain 3 No	1 Not important 2 Somewhat important 3 Very important

5. Should individuals within the organization who are not directly part of the care team have their incentives and responsibilities changed in order for the restructured care process to be effective? Can these changes be implemented?

References

General

Ahmann, E. "Family-Centered Care: Shifting Orientation." *Pediatric Nursing,* 1994, 20(2), 113–117.

Aiken, L. H., and others. "The Contribution of Specialists to the Delivery of Primary Care: A New Perspective." *New England Journal of Medicine,* 1979, 300(24), 1363–1370.

American Society of Internal Medicine. "Patient Access to Internist-Subspecialists in Gatekeeper Health Plans." Recommendations of the American Society of Internal Medicine, Washington, D.C., Aug. 1995.

Ammerman, A. S., and others. "Nutrition Education for Cardiovascular Disease Prevention Among Low Income Population—Description and Pilot Evaluation of a Physician-Based Model." *Patient Education and Counseling,* 1992, 19, 5–18.

Argote, L. "Input Uncertainty and Organizational Coordination in Hospital Emergency Units." *Administrative Science Quarterly,* 1982, 27, 420–434.

Berwick, D. M., Baker, M. W., and Kramer, E. "The State of Quality Management in HMOs." *HMO Practice,* 1992, 6(1), 26–32.

Bettenhausen, K. L. "Five Years of Groups Research: What We Have Learned and What Needs to Be Addressed." *Journal of Management,* 1991, 17(2), 345–381.

Bishop, K. K., Woll, J., and Arango, P. *Family/Professional Collaboration for Children with Special Health Needs and Their Families.* Burlington: Department of Social Work, University of Vermont, 1993.

Braunwald, E. "Subspecialists and Internal Medicine: A Perspective." *Annals of Internal Medicine,* 1991, 114, 76–78.

Brody, D. S. "The Patient's Role in Clinical Decision-Making." *Annals of Internal Medicine,* 1980, 93, 718–722.

Brown, T. M. "An Historical View of Health Care Teams." In G. J. Agich (ed.), *Responsibility in Health Care.* Dordrecht, Holland: Reidel, 1982.

Burns, L. R., and Becker, S. W. "Leadership and Decision Making." In S. M. Shortell and A. D. Kaluzny (eds.), *Health Care Management: A Text in Organization Theory and Behavior.* New York: Wiley, 1983.

Campbell, J. D., Mauksch, H. O., Neikirk, H. J., and Hosokawa, M. C. "Collaborative Practice and Provider Styles of Delivering Health Care." *Social Science Medicine,* 1990, 30(12), 1359–1365.

Carew, D. K., Parisi-Carew, E., and Blanchard, K. H. "Group Development and Situational Leadership: A Model for Managing Groups." *Training and Development Journal,* June 1986, pp. 46–50.

Charns, M. P. "Work Design." In S. M. Shortell and A. D. Kaluzny (eds.), *Health Care Management: A Text in Organization Theory and Behavior.* New York: Wiley, 1983.

Charns, M. P., and Schaefer, M. J. "Environment." In *Health Care Organizations: A Model for Management.* Upper Saddle River, N.J.: Prentice Hall, 1983.

Chilingerian, J. A., and Glavin, M.P.V. "Temporary Firms in Community Hospitals: Elements of a Managerial Theory of Clinical Efficiency." *Medical Care Review,* 1994, 51(3), 289–335.

Christianson, J. B., and others. "Implementing Programs for Chronic Illness Management: The Case of Hypertension Services." *The Joint Commission Journal on Quality Improvement,* 1997, 23(11), 593–601.

Christakis, N. A., Jacobs, J. A., and Messikomer, C. M. "Change in Self-Definition from Specialist to Generalist in a National Sample of Physicians." *Annals of Internal Medicine,* 1994, 121(9), 669–675.

Conrad, P. "The Experience of Illness: Recent and New Directions." *Research in the Sociology of Health Care,* 1987, 196, 1–31.

Corbin, J. M., and Strauss, A. "Accompaniments of Chronic Illness: Changes in Body, Self, Biography and Biographical Time." *Research in the Sociology of Health Care,* 1987, 16, 249–281.

Corbin, J. M., and Strauss, A. "A Nursing Model for Chronic Illness Management Based upon the Trajectory Framework." *Scholarly Inquiry for Nursing Practice,* 1991, 5(3), 155–174.

Council on Graduate Medical Education. *Third Report: Improving Access to Health Care Through Physician Workforce Reform: Directions for the Twenty-First Century.* Washington, D.C.: U.S. Department of Health and Human Services, 1992.

Cunningham, R. "Mapping Boundaries Between Specialist and Primary Care." *Medicine and Health: Perspectives,* 1995, 49(37), 1–4.

Cunningham, R. "Disease Management Seeks to Duck Threat of
   'Balkanization.'" *Medicine and Health Perspectives*, 1997, *51*(27), 1–4.

David, F. R., Randolph, W. A., and Pearce, J. A., II. "Linking Technology and
   Structure to Enhance Group Performance." *Journal of Applied Psychology*,
   1989, *74*(2), 233–241.

Defino, T. "New Measures for Chronic Care." HMO *Magazine*, Sept.–Oct. 1995,
   pp. 23–26.

Dietrich, A. J., and others. "Do Primary Physicians Actually Manage Their
   Patients' Fee-for-Service Care?" *Journal of the American Medical Association*, 1988, *259*(21), 3145–3149.

Emanuel, E. J., and Emanuel, L. L. "Four Models of the Physician-Patient
   Relationship." *Journal of the American Medical Association*, 1992, *267*(16),
   2221–2226.

Evans, J. A. "The Role of the Nurse Manager in Creating an Environment for
   Collaborative Practice." *Holistic Nurse Practitioner*, 1994, *8*(3), 22–31.

Fishman, P., Von Korff, M., Lozano, P., and Itecht, J. "Chronic Care Costs in
   Managed Care." *Health Affairs*, 1997, *16*, 239–247.

Garrity, T. F. "Medical Compliance and the Clinician-Patient Relationship: A
   Review." *Social Science and Medicine, Part E, Medical Psychology*, 1981, *15*,
   215–222.

Gersick, C.J.G. "Time and Transition in Work Teams: Toward a New Model of
   Group Development." *Academy of Management Journal*, 1988, *31*(1), 9–41.

Gillick, M. "Is the Care of the Chronically Ill a Medical Prerogative?" *New
   England Journal of Medicine*, 1984, *310*(3), 190–193.

Gottlieb, L. K., Margolis, C. Z., and Schoenbaum, S. C. "Clinical Practice
   Guidelines at an HMO: Development and Implementation in a Quality
   Improvement Model." *Quality Review Bulletin*, Feb. 1990, pp. 80–86.

Greenfield, S., Kaplan, S., and Ware, J. E. "Expanding Patient Involvement in
   Care: Effects on Patient Outcomes." *Annals of Internal Medicine*, 1985,
   102, 520–528.

Greenwald, H. P., and others. "Interspecialty Variation in Office-Based Care."
   Medical Care, 1984, *22*(1), 14–29.

Hage, J. "Communication and Coordination." In S. M. Shortell and A. D.
   Kaluzny (eds.), *Health Care Management: A Text in Organization Theory
   and Behavior*. New York: Wiley, 1983.

Halstead, L. S. "Team Care in Chronic Illness: A Critical Review of the Literature of the Past Twenty-Five Years." *Archives of Physical Medicine Rehabilitation*, 1976, *57*, 507–511.

Hare, A. P. *Handbook of Small Group Research*. (2nd ed.) New York: Free Press,
   1976.

Haug, M. R., and Lavin, B. "Practitioner or Patient—Who's in Charge?" *Journal of Health and Social Behavior*, 1981, 22, 212–229.

Haynes, R. B., Wang, E., and Gomes, M. D. "A Critical Review of Interventions to Improve Compliance with Prescribed Medications." *Patient Education and Counseling*, 1987, 10, 155–166.

Hetherington, R. W., and Rundall, T. G. "The Social Structure of Work Groups." In S. M. Shortell and A. D. Kaluzny (eds.), *Health Care Management: A Text in Organization Theory and Behavior*. New York: Wiley, 1983.

Hoffman, C., and Rice, D. *Chronic Care in America: A Twenty-First Century Challenge*. Princeton, N.J.: Robert Wood Johnson Foundation, 1996.

Hoffman, C., Rice, D., and Sung, H-Y. "Persons with Chronic Conditions: Their Prevalence and Costs." *Journal of the American Medical Association*, 1996, 276(18), 1473–1479.

Institute of Medicine. *Definition of Primary Care*. Washington, D.C.: National Academy Press, 1994.

Jennings, B., Callahan, D., and Caplan, A. L. "Ethical Challenges of Chronic Illness." *Hastings Center Report*, 1988, suppl. 1, pp. 1–15.

Kassirer, J. P. "Access to Specialty Care." *New England Journal of Medicine*, 1994, 331(7), 1151–1153.

Keith, R. A. "The Comprehensive Treatment Team in Rehabilitation." *Archives of Physical Medicine Rehabilitation*, 1991, 72, 269–274.

Lacoursiere, R. B. *The Life Cycle of Groups: Group Development Stage Theory*. New York: Human Sciences Press, 1980.

Lefton, M., and Rosengren, W. R. "Organization and Clients: Lateral and Longitudinal Dimensions." *American Sociological Review*, 1966, 31, 802–810.

Lumsdon, K. "Disease Management: The Heat and Heartache over Retooling Patient Care Create Hard Choices." *Hospitals and Health Networks*, Apr. 5, 1995, pp. 34–36, 38, 42.

Marcenko, M., and Smith, L. K. "The Impact of Family-Centered Case Management Approach." *Social Work in Health Care*, 1992, 17(1), 87–101.

March, J., and Simon, H. *Organizations*. New York: Wiley, 1958.

McCann, D. P., and Blossom, H. J. "The Physician as a Patient Educator: From Theory to Practice." *Western Journal of Medicine*, 1990, 153(1), 44–49.

McEachern, J. E., Schiff, L., and Cogan, O. "How to Start a Direct Patient Care Team." *Quality Review Bulletin*, 1992, pp. 191–200.

McGrath, J. E. *Groups: Interaction and Performance*. Upper Saddle River, N.J.: Prentice Hall, 1984.

Medenhall, R. C., Moynihan, C. J., and Radecki, S. E. "The Relative Complexity of Primary Care Provided by Medical Specialists." *Medical Care*, 1984, 22(11), 987–1001.

Morisky, D. E., and others. "Evaluation of Family Health Education to Build Social Support for Long-Term Control of High Blood Pressure." *Health Education Quarterly*, 1985, 12(1), 35–50.

Mulley, A., Mendoza, G., Rockefeller, R., and Staker, L. "Involving Patients in Medical Decision Making." *Quality Connection*, 1996, 5(1), 5–7.

Nagi, S. Z. "Teamwork in Health Care in the US: A Sociological Perspective." *Health and Society/Milbank Memorial Fund Quarterly*, winter 1975, pp. 75–90.

Newhouse, J. "Patients at Risk: Health Reform and Risk Adjustment." *Health Affairs*, 1994, 13, 132–140.

Newton, J., Hayes, V., and Hutchinson, A. "Factors Influencing General Practitioners' Referral Decisions." *Family Practice*, 1991, 8(4), 308–313.

Parsons, T. "Suggestions for a Sociological Approach to the Theory of Organizations." In A. Etzioni (ed.), *Complex Organizations: A Sociological Reader*. Austin, Tex.: Holt, Rinehart and Winston, 1961.

Pawlson, L. G. "Chronic Illness: Implications of a New Paradigm for Health Care." *Journal on Quality Improvement*, 1994, 20(1), 33–39.

Pearce, J. A., II, and Ravlin, E. C. "The Design and Activation of Self-Regulating Work Groups." *Human Relations*, 1987, 40(11), 751–782.

Perrow, C. "A Framework for the Comparative Analysis of Organizations." *American Sociological Review*, 1967, 32(2), 194–207.

Peterson, C. "Disease Management: A Team Approach to Chronic Care." *HMO Magazine*, 1995, 36, 39–47.

Pigg, J. S. "Role of Nursing and Allied Health Professions in the Treatment of Arthritis." In D.H.J. McCarty (ed.), *Arthritis and Allied Conditions*. (11th ed.) Baltimore: Lea and Febiger, 1988.

Roberts, J., and others. "The Effectiveness and Efficiency of Health Promotion in Specialty Clinic Care." *Medical Care*, 1995, 33(9), 892–905.

Rummler, G. A., and Brache, A. P. *Improving Performance: How to Manage the White Space on an Organization Chart*. San Francisco: Jossey-Bass, 1995.

Russell, N., and Roter, D. "Health Promotion Counseling of Chronic-Disease Patients During Primary Care Visits." *American Journal of Public Health*, 1993, 83(7), 979–982.

Schellevis, F. G., and others. "Validity of Diagnoses of Chronic Diseases in General Practice." *Journal of Clinical Epidemiology*, 1993, 46(5), 461–468.

Schellevis, F. G., and others. "Implementing Guidelines in General Practice: Evaluation of Process and Outcome of Care in Chronic Diseases." *International Journal for Quality in Health Care*, 1994, 6(3), 257–266.

Schlesinger, M. "On the Limits of Expanding Health Care Reform: Chronic Care in Prepaid Settings." *Milbank Quarterly*, 1986, 64(2), 189–215.

Schlesinger, M., and Mechanic, D. "Challenges for Managed Competition from Chronic Illness." *Health Affairs*, 1993, suppl., pp. 124–137.

Shortell, S. M., and Kaluzny, A. D. (eds.). *Health Care Management: A Text in Organization Theory and Behavior*. New York: Wiley, 1983.

Speedling, E. J., and Rose, D. N. "Building an Effective Doctor-Patient Relationship: From Patient Satisfaction to Patient Participation." *Social Science Medicine*, 1985, *21*(2), 115–120.

Starfield, B. H., Simborg, D. W., Horn, S. D., and Yourtee, S. A. "Continuity and Coordination in Primary Care: Their Achievement and Utility." *Medical Care*, 1976, *14*(7), 625–636.

Strauss, A. L., Fagerhaugh, S., Suczek, B., and Wiener, C. *The Social Organization of Medical Work*. Chicago: University of Chicago Press, 1985.

Taylor, N. "Partnering with Disease State Management Vendors: Is It Risky Business?" *Quality Letter*, Nov. 1995, pp. 11–16.

Thompson, J. D. *Organizations in Action*. New York: McGraw-Hill, 1967.

Wagner, E. H., Austin, B. T., and Von Korff, M. "Organizing Care for Patients with Chronic Illness." *Milbank Quarterly*, 1996, *74*(4), 511–544.

Walker, E. A. "Shaping the Course of a Marathon: Using the Trajectory Framework for Diabetes Mellitus." *Scholarly Inquiry for Nursing Practice*, 1991, *5*(3), 235–242.

Wall, V. D., Galanes, G. J., and Love, S. B. "Small, Task-Oriented Groups: Conflict, Conflict Management, Satisfaction, and Decision Quality." *Small Group Behavior*, 1987, *18*(1), 31–55.

Wall, V. D., and Nolan, L. L. "Perceptions of Inequity, Satisfaction, and Conflict in Task-Oriented Groups." *Human Relations*, 1986, *39*(11), 1033–1052.

Wall, V. D., and Nolan, L. L. "Small Group Conflict: A Look at Equity, Satisfaction, and Styles of Conflict Management." *Small Group Behavior*, 1987, *18*(2), 188–211.

Walsh, J.M.E., and McPhee, S. J. "A Systems Model of Clinical Preventive Care: An Analysis of Factors Influencing Patient and Physician." *Health Education Quarterly*, 1992, *19*(2), 157–175.

Weel, C. V. "Teamwork." *Lancet*, 1994, *344*, 1276–1279.

Westbom, L., and Kornfält, R. "Utilization of Primary Care Versus Specialized Care in Children with and Without Chronic Illness." *Acta Paediatrica Scandinavica*, 1991, *80*, 534–541.

White, M., Gundrum, G., Shearer, S., and Simmons, W. J. "A Role for Case Managers in the Physician Office." *Journal of Case Management*, 1994, *3*(2), 62–68.

Williams, P. T. "The Role of Family Physicians in the Management of Cancer Patients." *Journal of Cancer Education*, 1994, *9*, 67–72.

Wise, D. "Tailormade Care." *HMO Magazine*, 1993, *34*(4), 24–29.

Zalta, E., Eichner, H., and Henry, M. "Implications of Disease Management in the Future of Managed Care." *Medical Interface*, Dec. 1994, pp. 66–78.

Asthma

Bailey, W. C., and others. "A Randomized Trial to Improve Self-Management Practices of Adults with Asthma." *Archives of Internal Medicine*, 1990, *150*, 1664–1668.

Blancquaert, I. R., Zvagulis, I., Gray-Donald, K., and Pless, I. B. "Referral Patterns for Children with Chronic Diseases." *Pediatrics*, 1992, *90*, 71–74.

Boner, A. L., and Valletta, E. A. "Education in Asthmatic Children." *Monaldi Archives of Chest Disease*, 1994, *49*(3), 250–253.

Centers for Disease Control. "Asthma: United States, 1982–1992." *Morbidity and Mortality Weekly Report*, 1995, *326*, 862.

Charlton, I., Charlton, G., Broomfield, J., and Campbell, M. "An Evaluation of a Nurse-Run Asthma Clinic in General Practice Using an Attitudes and Morbidity Questionnaire." *Family Practice*, 1992, *9*(2), 154–160.

Charlton, I., Charlton, G., Broomfield, J., and Mullee, M. A. "Audit of the Effect of a Nurse Run Asthma Clinic on Workload and Patient Morbidity in a General Practice." *British Journal of General Practice*, 1991, *41*, 227–231.

Engel, W., Freund, D. A., Stein, J. S., and Fletcher, R. H. "The Treatment of Patients with Asthma by Specialists and Generalists." *Medical Care*, 1989, *27*, 306–314.

Evans, R., and others. "National Trends in the Morbidity and Mortality of Asthma in the U.S." *Chest*, 1987, *91*, suppl. 6, 65S–74S.

Freund, D. A., and others. "Specialty Differences in the Treatment of Asthma." *Journal of Allergy and Clinical Immunology*, 1989, pp. 401–406.

Greineder, D. K., Loane, K. C., and Parks, P. "Reduction in Resource Utilization by an Asthma Outreach Program." *Archives of Pediatric and Adolescent Medicine*, 1995, *149*, 415–420.

Hughes, D. M., McLeod, M., Garner, B., and Goldbloom, R. B. "Controlled Trial of a Home and Ambulatory Program for Asthmatic Children." *Pediatrics*, 1991, *87*, 54–61.

Kretz, S. E., and Meyer, L. C. "Improving Patient Outcomes for Severe Asthma Through Comprehensive, Specialized Treatment." Report summary. Denver: National Jewish Center for Immunology and Respiratory Medicine and the John Hancock Mutual Life Insurance Company, 1993.

Lewis, C. E., and others. "A Randomized Trial of A.C.T. (Asthma Care Training) for Kids." *Pediatrics*, 1984, *74*, 478–486.

Mason, R. J., Katz, J. L., and Bethel, R. A. "Time Out for Asthma: Rationale for a Comprehensive Evaluation." *Seminars in Respiratory and Critical Care Medicine*, 1994, *15*(2), 97–105.

Mayo, P. H., Richman, J., and Harris, H. W. "Results of a Program to Reduce Admissions for Adult Asthma." *Annals of Internal Medicine*, 1990, *112*, 864–871.

Miller, B. D., and Wood, B. L. "Childhood Asthma in Interaction with Family, School and Peer Systems: A Developmental Model for Primary Care." *Journal of Asthma*, 1991, *28*, 405–414.

Rohl, B. J., Meyer, L. C., and Lung, C. L. "An Individualized, Comprehensive Asthma Care Treatment Program." *Asthma Care*, Mar. 1994, pp. 121–123, 134.

Stevens, M. A., and Weiss-Harrison, A. "A Program for Children with Asthma." *HMO Practice*, 1993, *7*(2), 91–93.

Todd, W. E. "New Mindsets in Asthma: Interventions and Disease Management." *The Journal of Care Management*, 1995, *1*, 1–8.

van Damme, R., Drummond, N., Beattie, J., and Douglas, G. "Integrated Care for Patients with Asthma: Views of General Practitioners." *British Journal of General Practice*, 1994, *44*(378), 9–13.

Weiss, K. B., Gergen, P. J., and Hodgson, T. A. "An Economic Evaluation of Asthma in the United States." *New England Journal of Medicine*, 1992, *326*, 862–866.

Wilson, S. R., and others. "A Controlled Trial of Two Forms of Self-Management Education for Adults with Asthma." *American Journal of Medicine*, 1993, *94*, 564–576.

Windsor, R. A., and others. "Evaluation of the Efficacy and Cost Effectiveness of Health Education Methods to Increase Medication Adherence Among Adults with Asthma." *American Journal of Public Health*, 1990, 80(12), 1519–1521.

Zablocki, E. "A Breath of Fresh Air." *HMO Magazine*, May–June 1995, pp. 51–57.

Zieger, R. S., and others. "Facilitated Referral to Asthma Specialist Reduces Relapses in Asthma Emergency Room Visits." *Journal of Allergy and Clinical Immunology*, 1991, *87*, 1160–1168.

Arthritis

Ahlmen, M., Bjelle, A., and Sullivan, M. "Prediction of Team Care Effects in Outpatients with Rheumatoid Arthritis." *Journal of Rheumatology*, 1991, *18*, 1655–1661.

Ahlmen, M., Sullivan, M., and Bjelle, A. "Team Versus Non-Team Outpatient Care in Rheumatoid Arthritis." *Arthritis and Rheumatism*, 1988, *31*, 471–479.

American Nurses' Association. *Outcome Standards for Rheumatology Nursing Practice*. Kansas City: American Nurses' Association, 1983.

Ansell, B. M. "How Should Pediatric Rheumatology Be Delivered?" *Clinical and Experimental Rheumatology*, 1994, *12*, S113–S116.

Bilodeau, A. "In a New Pilot Project, HMO Patients and Physicians Are Learning How to Manage Arthritis Pain from People Who Know Best—Arthritis Patients." *HMO Magazine*, July–Aug. 1995, pp. 71–74.

Duff, I. F., Carpenter, J. O., and Neukom, J. E. "Comprehensive Management of Patients with Rheumatoid Arthritis: Some Results of the Regional Arthritis Control Program in Michigan." *Arthritis and Rheumatism*, 1974, *17*, 635–645.

Goeppinger, J., and others. "A Reexamination of the Effectiveness of Self-Care Education for Persons with Arthritis." *Arthritis and Rheumatism*, 1989, *32*, 706–716.

Hughes, R. B., and D'Ambrosia, K. "Nursing Management of a Child with Juvenile Rheumatoid Arthritis." *Orthopaedic Nursing*, 1993, *12*, 17–22.

Lorig, K. R., and Holman, H. "Arthritis Self-Management Studies: A Twelve-Year Review." *Health Education Quarterly*, 1993, *12*, 17–28.

Lorig, K., Konkol, L., and Gonzalez, V. "Arthritis Patient Education: A Review of the Literature." *Patient Education and Counseling*, 1987, *10*, 207–252.

Lorig, K. R., Mazonson, P. D., and Holman, H. R. "Evidence Suggesting That Health Education for Self-Management in Patients with Chronic Arthritis Has Sustained Health Benefits While Reducing Health Care Costs." *Arthritis and Rheumatism*, 1993, *36*, 439–446.

Lorig, K., and others. "Outcomes of Self-Help Education for Patients with Arthritis." *Arthritis and Rheumatism*, 1985, *28*, 680–685.

Lorig, K., and others. *Living a Healthy Life with Chronic Conditions*. Palo Alto, Calif.: Bull, 1994.

Lynch, N. M., and Caughey, D. E. "Team Management of Chronic Arthritis." *Journal of Rheumatology*, 1995, *22*, 1005–1006.

Mullen, P. D., Laville, E. A., Biddle, A. K., and Lorig, K. "Efficacy of Psychoeducational Interventions on Pain, Depression, and Disability in People with Arthritis: A Meta-Analysis." *Journal of Rheumatology*, 1987, *15*, 33–39.

Neuberger, G. B., Smith, K. V., Black, S. O., and Hassanein, R. "Promoting Self-Care in Clients with Arthritis." *Arthritis Care and Research*, 1993, *6*, 141–148.

Pigg, J. S., Driscoll, P. W., and Caniff, R. *Rheumatology Nursing: A Problem Oriented Approach*. New York: Wiley, 1985.

Rapoff, M. A., Lindsley, C. B., and Christophersen, E. R. "Parent Perceptions of Problems Experienced by Their Children in Complying with Treatments for Juvenile Rheumatoid Arthritis." *Archives of Physical Medicine and Rehabilitation*, 1985, 66, 427–430.

Raspe, H. H., Deck, R., and Mattussek, S. "The Outcome of Traditional or Comprehensive Outpatient Care for Rheumatoid Arthritis (RA)." *Zeitschrift fur Rheumatologie*, 1992, 51, suppl. 1, 61–66.

Schned, E. S., and others. "Team Managed Outpatient Care for Early Onset of Chronic Inflammatory Arthritis." *Journal of Rheumatology*, 1995, 22, 1141–1148.

Verbrugge, L. M., and Patrick, D. L. "Seven Chronic Conditions: Their Impact on U.S. Adults' Activity Levels and Use of Medical Services." *American Journal of Public Health*, 1995, 85, 173–182.

Wiener, C. L. "The Burden of Rheumatoid Arthritis: Tolerating the Uncertainty." *Social Science and Medicine*, 1975, 9, 97–104.

Yelin, E. "Arthritis: The Cumulative Impact of a Chronic Condition." *Arthritis and Rheumatism*, 1992, 35, 489–497.

Diabetes

American Diabetes Association (ADA). *Diabetes: 1993 Vital Statistics*. Alexandria, Va.: American Diabetes Association, 1993.

Bild, D. E., and others. "Lower Extremity Amputation in People with Diabetes." *Diabetes Care*, 1989, 12, 24–31.

Boucher, B. J., and others. "A Pilot Support Service Based on Family Practice Attenders: Comparison with Diabetic Clinics in East London." *Diabetic Medicine*, 1987, 4, 480–484.

British Multicentre Study Group. "Proliferative Diabetic Retinopathy; Treatment with Xenon-Arc Photocoagulation." *British Medical Journal*, 1977, 1, 739–741.

Carlson, A., and Rosenqvist, U. "Diabetes Control Program Implementation: On the Importance of Staff Involvement." *Scandinavian Journal of Primary Health Care*, 1988, suppl. 1, pp. 105–112.

Comi, R. J. "A Unique Collaborative Network for Diabetes Education." *Diabetes Educator*, 1991, 17(6), 442–445.

Day, J. L., Metcalfe, J., and Johnson, P. "Benefits Provided by an Integrated Education and Clinical Diabetes Center: A Follow-Up Study." *Diabetic Medicine*, 1992, 9(9), 855–859.

Drash, A. L. "Clinical Care of the Patient with Diabetes: What Is the Role of the Diabetes Professional?" *Diabetes Care*, 1994, *17*, suppl. 1, 40–44.

Etzwiler, D. D. "The Patient Is a Member of the Medical Team." *Journal of the American Dietetic Association*, 1972, *61*, 421–423.

Funnell, M. M., and others. "Empowerment: An Idea Whose Time Has Come in Diabetes Education." *Diabetes Educator*, 1991, *17*(1), 37–41.

Gewirtz, G. "Current Thoughts on Diabetes Patient Education in New Jersey." *New Jersey Medicine*, 1994, *91*(4), 230–232.

Gibbons, R. L., and Saunders, J. "How to Do It: Develop Diabetic Care in General Practice." *British Medical Journal*, 1988, *297*, 187–189.

Gonen, B., and Horwitz, D. I. "Haemoglobin A$_1$: An Indicator of the Metabolic Control of Diabetic Patients." *Lancet*, 1977, *2*, 734–737.

Hayes, T. M., and Harries, J. "Randomized Controlled Trial of Routine Hospital Clinic Care Versus Routine General Practice Care for Type II Diabetics." *British Medical Journal*, 1984, *289*, 728–730.

Hiss, R. G. (ed.). *Diabetes in Communities*. Ann Arbor: University of Michigan, 1986.

Koperski, M. "How Effective Is Systematic Care of Diabetic Patients? A Study in One General Practice." *British Journal of General Practice*, 1992, *42*, 508–511.

Kronsbein, P., and others. "Evaluation of a Structured Treatment and Teaching Programme on Non-Insulin-Dependent Diabetes." *Lancet*, Dec. 1988, pp. 1407–1411.

Lyon, R. B., and Vinci, D. M. "Nutrition Management of Insulin-Dependent Diabetes Mellitus in Adults: Review by the Diabetes Care and Education Dietetic Practice Group." *Journal of the American Dietetic Association*, 1993, *93*(3), 309–314.

Mann, N. P., and Johnston, D. I. "Total Glycosylated Haemoglobin Levels in Diabetic Children." *Archives of Disease in Children*, 1982, *57*(6), 434–437.

Mazze, R. S., Bergenstal, R., and Ginsberg, B. "Intensified Diabetes Management: Lessons from the Diabetes Control and Complications Trial." *International Journal of Clinical Pharmacology and Therapeutics*, 1995, *33*(1), 43–51.

Mazze, R. S., and others. "Staged Diabetes Management: Toward an Integrated Model of Diabetes Care." *Diabetes Care*, 1994, suppl. 1, *17*(1), 56–66.

McDonald, G. W. "Diabetes Supplement of the National Health Survey." *Journal of the American Dietetic Association*, 1968, *52*, 118.

McLemoe, T., and Delozier, J. *Summary: National Ambulatory Medical Care Survey—Advance Data from Vital and Health Statistics, 1987*. Department

of Health and Human Services publication no. (PHS) 87–1250.
Hyattsville, Md.: National Center for Health Statistics, U.S. Department
of Health and Human Services, 1987.

Parving, H.-H., and Hommel, E. "Prognosis in Diabetic Nephropathy." *British
Medical Journal*, 1989, 299, 230–233.

Peterson, K. A. "Diabetes Care by Primary Care Physicians in Minnesota and
Wisconsin." *Journal of Family Practice*, 1994, 38(4), 361–367.

Rifkin, H., and Porte, D. (eds.). *Diabetes Mellitus: Theory and Practice*. (4th ed.)
New York: Elsevier, 1990.

Rosenqvist, U., Carlson, A., and Luft, R. "Evaluation of Comprehensive
Program for Diabetes Care at Primary Health Care Level." *Diabetes Care*,
1988, 11(3), 269–274.

Siddons, H., and McAughey, D. "Professional Development Brings Specialist
Knowledge: The Role of the Diabetes Specialist Nurse—The Manchester
Model." *Professional Nurse*, 1992, 7(5), 321–324.

Tattersall, R. B., and McMulloch, D. K. "Modern Aspects of Conventional
Insulin Therapy." *Annals of Clinical Research*, 1984, 16, 107–117.

Walker, E. A. "Shaping the Course of a Marathon: Using the Trajectory Framework for Diabetes Mellitus." *Scholarly Inquiry for Nursing Practice*, 1991,
5(3), 235–242, 243–248 (discussion section).

Weinberger, M., and others. "A Nurse-Coordinated Intervention for Primary
Care Patients with Non-Insulin-Dependent Diabetes Mellitus." *Journal
of General Internal Medicine*, 1995, 10, 59–65.

Hypertension

Adamson, T. E., Rodnick, J. E., and Guillion, D. S. "Family Physicians and
General Internists: Do They Treat Hypertensive Patients Differently?"
Journal of Family Practice, 1989, 29(1), 93–99.

Applegate, W. B. "Managing the Older Patient with Hypertension." *American
Journal of Hypertension*, 1993, 6, 277S–282S.

Burt, V. L., and others. "Prevalence of Hypertension in the U.S. Adult Population." *Hypertension*, 1995, 25, 305–313.

Chalmers, J., and Zanchetti, A. "The 1996 Report of a World Health Organization Expert Committee on Hypertension Control." *Journal of Hypertension*, 1996, 14, 929–933.

Davis, B., and others. "Lack of Effectiveness of a Low-Sodium/High-Potassium
Diet in Reducing Antihypertensive Medication Requirements in
Overweight Persons with Mild Hypertension." *American Journal of
Hypertension*, 1994, 7, 926–932.

Degoulet, P., and others. "Factors Predictive of Attendance at Clinic and Blood Pressure Control in Hypertensive Patients." *British Medical Journal*, 1983, 287, 88–93.

Dickinson, J. C., and others. "Improving Hypertension Control: Impact of Computer Feedback and Physician Education." *Medical Care*, 1981, 19(8), 843–854.

Farmer, K. C., Jacobs, E. W., and Phillips, C. R. "Long-Term Patient Compliance with Prescribed Regimens of Calcium Channel Blockers." *Clinical Therapy*, 1994, 16(2), 316–326.

Foote, A., and Erfurt, J. C. "The Benefit to Cost Ratio of Work-Site Blood Pressure Control Programs." *Journal of the American Medical Association*, 1991, 265, 1238–1286.

Greenfield, S., and others. "Outcomes of Patients with Hypertension and Non-Insulin-Dependent Diabetes Mellitus Treated by Different Systems and Specialties." *Journal of the American Medical Association*, 1995, 274, 1436–1444.

Harris, L. E., Luft, F. C., Rudy, D. W., and Tierney, W. M. "Correlates of Health Care Satisfaction in Inner-City Patients with Hypertension and Chronic Renal Insufficiency." *Social Science and Medicine*, 1995, 41(12), 1639–1645.

Healthy People 2000. *National Health Promotion and Disease Prevention Objectives*. Department of Health and Human Services publication no. (PHS) 91–50212. Hyattsville, Md.: National Center for Health Statistics, U.S. Department of Health and Human Services, 1991.

Heurtin-Roberts, S., and Reisin, E. "The Relation of Culturally Influenced Lay Models of Hypertension to Compliance with Treatment." *American Journal of Hypertension*, 1992, 5(11), 787–792.

Krakoff, L. R. "Ambulatory Blood Pressure Monitoring Can Improve Cost-Effective Management of Hypertension." *American Journal of Hypertension*, 1993, 6(22), 220S–224S.

Levine, D. M., Green, L. W., and Morisky, D. "Effect of a Structures Health Education Program on Reducing Morbidity and Mortality from High Blood Pressure." *Bibliotheca Cardiologica*, 1987, 42, 8–16.

Levy, D., and others. "The Progression from Hypertension to Congestive Heart Failure." *Journal of the American Medical Association*, 1996, 275(20), 1557–1562.

Lüscher, T. F., Vetter, H., Siegenthaler, W., and Vetter, W. "Compliance in Hypertension: Facts and Concepts." *Journal of Hypertension*, 1985, 3, suppl. 1, 3–9.

MacMahon, S. "Guidelines for Antihypertensive Therapy." *Journal of Hypertension*, 1996, *14*, 691–693.

Menard, J., and Chatellier, G. "Limiting Factors in the Control of BP: Why Is There a Gap Between Theory and Practice?" *Journal of Human Hypertension*, 1995, 9(2), S19–S23.

Morisky, D. E., and others. "Five-Year Blood Pressure Control and Mortality Following Health Education for Hypertensive Patients." *American Journal of Public Health*, 1983, 73(2), 153–162.

National Center for Health Statistics. *Current Estimates from the National Health Interview Survey, 1994.* Department of Health and Human Services publication no. (PHS) 96–1421. Hyattsville, Md.: National Center for Health Statistics, U.S. Department of Health and Human Services, 1994.

Oberman, A., and others. "Pharmacologic and Nutritional Treatment of Mild Hypertension: Changes in Cardiovascular Risk Status." *Annals of Internal Medicine*, 1990, *111*, 89–95.

Richardson, M. A., Simons-Morton, B., and Annegers, J. F. "Effect of Perceived Barriers on Compliance with Antihypertensive Medication." *Health Education Quarterly*, 1993, 20(4), 489–503.

Savage, D. D., McGee, D. L., and Oster, G. "Reduction of Hypertension-Associated Heart Disease and Stroke Among Black Americans: Past Experience and New Perspectives on Targeting Resources." *Milbank Quarterly*, 1987, 65(2), 297–321.

Schmieder, R. E., Rockstroh, J. K., and Messerli, F. H. "Antihypertensive Therapy: To Stop or Not to Stop?" *Journal of the American Medical Association*, 1991, *265*, 1566–1571.

Schultz, F. J., and Sheps, S. G. "Management of Patients with Hypertension: A Hypertension Clinic Model." *Mayo Clinic Proceedings*, 1994, *69*, 997–999.

Stamler, R., and others. "Primary Prevention of Hypertension by Nutritional-Hygienic Means: Final Report of a Randomized, Controlled Trial." *Journal of the American Medical Association*, 1989, *262*, 1801–1807.

Treatment of Mild Hypertension Research Group. "The Treatment of Mild Hypertension Study: A Randomized, Placebo-Controlled Trial of a Nutritional-Hygienic Regimen Along with Various Drug Monotherapies." *Archives of Internal Medicine*, 1991, *151*, 1413–1423.

Whelton, P. K., and Brancati, F. L. "Hypertension Management in Populations." *Clinical and Experimental Hypertension*, 1993, *15*(6), 1147–1156.

Stable Coronary Artery Disease

American Heart Association. *1990 Heart and Stroke Facts.* Dallas: American Heart Association, 1990.

American Heart Association. *1994 Heart and Stroke Facts Statistics*. Dallas: American Heart Association, 1993.

Carbajal, E. V., and Deedwania, P. C. "Contemporary Approaches in Medical Management of Patients with Stable Coronary Artery Disease." *Medical Clinics in North America*, 1995, 79(5), 1063–1084.

Centers for Disease Control and Prevention. "Estimated National Spending on Prevention: United States, 1988." *Morbidity and Mortality Weekly Report*, 1992, 41, 529–531.

Deedwania, P., and Carbajal, E. "Silent Ischemia During Daily Life Is an Independent Predictor of Mortality in Stable Angina." *Circulation*, 1990, 81, 748–756.

Frye, R. L., and others. "Treatment of Coronary Artery Disease." *Journal of the American College of Cardiology*, 1989, 13(5), 957–968.

Gillum, R. "Trends in Acute Myocardial Infarction and Coronary Artery Disease Death in the United States." *Journal of the American College of Cardiology*, 1993, 23, 1273–1277.

Gillum, R., Folsom, A., and Blackburn, H. "The Decline in Coronary Artery Disease Mortality: Old Questions and New Facts." *American Journal of Medicine*, 1984, 76, 1055–1065.

Healthy People 2000. *National Health Promotion and Disease Prevention Objectives*. Department of Health and Human Services publication no. (PHS) 91–50212. Hyattsville, Md.: National Center for Health Statistics, U.S. Department of Health and Human Services, 1991.

Institute for Clinical Systems Integration (ICSI). *Health Care Guideline: Stable Coronary Artery Disease*. Minneapolis: Institute for Clinical Systems Integration, 1995.

Kingsley, C. M., and Gupta, S. C. "How to Reduce the Risk of Coronary Artery Disease: Teaching Patients a Healthy Life-Style." *Postgraduate Medicine*, 1992, 91(4), 147–160.

Mullen, P. D., Mains, D. A., and Velez, R. "A Meta-Analysis of Controlled Trials of Cardiac Patient Education." *Patient Education and Counseling*, 1992, 19, 143–162.

Parchert, M., and Simon, J. "The Role of Exercise in Cardiac Rehabilitation: A Nursing Perspective." *Rehabilitative Nursing*, 1988, 12, 11.

Rocco, M., and others. "Prognostic Importance of Myocardial Ischemia Detected by Ambulatory Monitoring in Patients with Stable Coronary Artery Disease." *Circulation*, 1988, 78, 877–884.

Stern, S., and Tzivoni, D. "Early Detection of Silent Ischemic Heart Disease by Twenty-Four Hour Electrocardiographic Monitoring of Active Subjects." *British Heart Journal*, 1974, 36, 481–486.

Stovsky, B. "Nursing Interventions for Risk Factor Reduction." *Nursing Clinics of North America*, 1992, 27(1), 257–269.

Tzivoni, D., and others. "Comparison of Mortality and Myocardial Infarction Rates in Stable Angina Pectoris with and Without Ischemic Episodes During Daily Activities." *American Journal of Cardiology*, 1989, 63, 273–276.

Yates, B. C. "The Relationships Among Social Support and Short- and Long-Term Recovery Outcomes in Men with Coronary Heart Disease." *Research in Nursing and Health*, 1995, 18, 193–203.

Name Index

216   Name Index

Meyer, K. R., 100, 114, 116–117
Meyer, L. C., 22, 25
Miller, B. D., 26
Morisky, D. E., 16, 43
Moynihan, C. J., 13
Mullee, M. A., 22–23
Mullen, P. D., 30, 47
Mulley, A., 11

N

Nagi, S. Z., 19
National Center for Health Statistics, 41
Neikirk, H. J., 14
Neuberger, G. B., 29
Neukom, J. E., 31
Newhouse, J., 6
Newton, J., 13
Nolan, L. L., 59

O

Oberman, 44
Oster, G., 40

P

Paquette, M. P., 94, 114–115, 121, 123–125
Parchert, M., 48
Parisi-Carew, E., 75–78
Parks, P., 22
Parsons, T., 54
Parving, H.-H., 33
Patrick, D. L., 28
Pawlson, L. G., 3
Pearce, J. A., II, 61, 70
Perrow, C., 53
Peterson, C., 2
Phillips, C. R., 43
Pigg, J. S., 14, 97, 115, 117–118, 128
Pless, I. B., 24
Porte, D., 33

R

Radecki, S. E., 13
Randolph, W. A., 61
Rapoff, M. A., 32
Raspe, H. H., 31

Ravlin, E. C., 70
Reisin, E., 43
Rice, D., 1, 5
Richardson, M. A., 43
Richman, J., 22
Rifkin, H., 33
Roberts, J., 149
Rocco, M., 46
Rockefeller, R., 11
Rockstroh, J. K., 42
Rodnick, J. E., 44
Rohl, B. J., 25
Rose, D. N., 6, 11
Rosenqvist, U., 35, 36
Roter, D., 6
Rudy, D. W., 41
Rummler, G. A., 162
Rundall, T. G., 54–55, 56, 58, 60, 80
Russell, N., 6

S

Saunders, J., 36
Savage, D. D., 40
Schaefer, M. J., 79, 80–81, 84, 85
Schellevis, F. G., 6, 12
Schlesinger, M., 16
Schmieder, R. E., 42
Schned, E. S., 31, 32, 33
Schoenbaum, S. C., 83
Schultz, F. J., 45
Selby, J., 105, 115, 120, 122, 123, 128
Shearer, S., 14
Sheps, S. G., 45
Shortell, S. M., 59
Siddons, H., 35
Siegenthaler, W., 43
Simborg, D. W., 17
Simmons, W. J., 14
Simon, H. 58, 79
Simon, J., 48
Simons-Morton, B., 43
Smith, K. V., 29
Smith, L. K., 16
Speedling, E. J., 6, 11
Staker, L., 11

Subject Index